the salt spring experience

We dedicate this book to Baba Hari Dass, our spiritual teacher, without whom there would be no Salt Spring Centre . . . and no book.

the salt spring experience

recipes for body, mind, and spirit

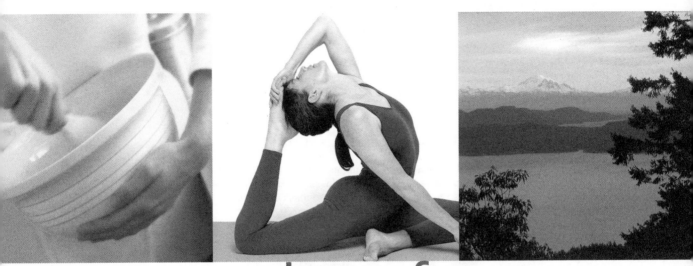

FROM THE SALT SPRING CENTRE

MACMILLIAN CANADA
TORONTO

First published in Canada in 2001 by
Macmillan Canada, an imprint of CDG Books Canada Inc.

National Library of Canada Cataloguing in Publication Data

The Salt Spring Centre
        The Salt Spring experience : recipes for body, mind and spirit

Includes index.
ISBN 1-55335-009-X

1. Vegetarian cookery. 2. Yoga, Hatha. 3. Holistic medicine.
I. Title.
TX837.F44 2001   641.5'636   C2001-901655-7

This book is available at special discounts for bulk purchases by your group
or organization for sales promotions, premiums, fundraising and seminars.
For details, contact: CDG Books Canada Inc., 99 Yorkville Avenue, Suite 400,
Toronto, ON, M5R 3K5. Tel: 416-963-8830. Toll Free: 1-877-963-8830.
Fax: 416-923-4821. Web site: cdgbooks.com.

1 2 3 4 5 KRO 05 04 03 02 01

Cover and text design by Carol Moskot
Photography by Derrick Lundy and Osman Phillips
Cover food photo by Burazin/Masterfile

Macmillan Canada
An imprint of CDG Books Canada Inc.
Toronto

Printed in Canada

acknowledgements

Authors: Sharada Filkow and Mayana Williamson

Ayurveda chapter: Cynthia Ambika Copple

Asana teachers and consultants: Celeste Aradhana Mallett and Andrea Kalpana Tabachnick

Recipe development and testing: Sharada Filkow (coordinator), Ramanand Chlopan, Mary Conrad, Sid Filkow, Scott Fotheringham, Krista Whaley

Photography: Derrick Lundy—colour insert, black and white (other than asana chapter) front cover (nature); Osman Phillips—Asana chapter, front cover (asana), and back cover (author photo)

Asana models: Rick Abramyk, Celeste Aradhana Mallett, and Andrea Kalpana Tabachnick

Makeup and hair styling for asana photos: Lyndsay Savage

We appreciate the helpfulness and generosity of the following people:

Thank you to Bhavani Siegel for help with the asana chapter, Jennifer Radhika Charles for help with the Spirit of Play chapter, Rajani Rock for the Fragrant Flower Facial, Gail Bryn-Jones for the Virtues Acknowledgement, Mouat's Trading Company for asana props, and to Susan Lundy and Driftwood Publishing for use of their office and transmission of image files. Thank you to Pamela Thornley for food research and her ever-present sense of humour, and to Sharon Jeevani Sorrell for recipe typing and loving encouragement.

Thank you to Jennifer Lambert, our editor, for skill and clarity, for the ability to make stressful events seem manageable, and for her quietly enthusiastic support at every stage of the project.

Thank you to our Centre family for consistent support and encouragement, and for always being there.

contents

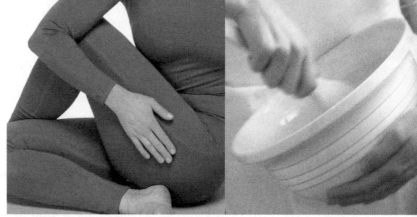

foreword by david wood

FEW OF US WHO LIVE ON SALT SPRING WERE BORN HERE; almost everyone is from some-where else and made a conscious choice to come. There are many reasons why people come—to live on an island with a gentle climate, but still in Canada; to live in a small community where you can be on smiling terms with a good part of the population; to have a general, easy acceptance of one another in a place with remarkable diversity; to live closer to nature and be surrounded by truly stunning natural beauty; or to enjoy that pleasant mix of small town and rural living that makes for a safe and lovely place to bring up children. All these factors play a role, small or large, in each of our decisions to come to Salt Spring. They are the common ground that we share, and when passionate disagreements on local issues periodically threaten to tear us apart, they are the glue that holds us together. The common theme that runs through all of us, whether we are con-scious of it or not, is the desire to find peace. We strive to find more peace in our lives and in our-selves than we were able to find wherever it was that we lived before.

It is certainly true with my family. We came to Salt Spring from Toronto, where, from the outside, we lived the life that comes with a seemingly successful small business in the city. But, as is always the case, the way it looked from the outside did not convey the reality of what it was like on the inside. Even superficially, it was a divided life: I spent all my time working, and Nancy, my wife, spent all her time taking care of the children. There was very little overlap between the two. We also had the beginnings of middle-aged angst, when the rewards that you have struggled for begin to pall and you start thinking there has to be more to life. We dimly realized, although at the time we were not brave enough to admit it to our friends and families, that we had started to look for the missing element; we were lucky enough to choose Salt Spring Island as the place to do it.

You cannot be very long on the island without becoming aware of the Salt Spring Centre. It occupies a beautiful piece of property in the middle of the island and houses a small commu-nity of followers of Baba Hari Dass, a yogi, monk, and accomplished scholar. To an outsider, they seemed a close-knit, somewhat alternative group. I felt as I remember feeling about the Rolling Stones in my early 20s: that these people had something I envied, but I doubted that

I could ever let go enough to have a chance of getting some of it for myself.

And there matters would probably have rested, had not one of our children run into trouble at school. Josh, a bright 10-year-old, had been diagnosed with quite severe learning disabilities. It was difficult for him to keep up with his class and it was demolishing his self-esteem. Friends suggested the Salt Spring Centre School. It had a reputation for providing an education where the child came first. We reckoned that if they could rekindle Josh's love of learning he would be able to learn the curriculum, and a lot more besides, when he needed to. And that is exactly what happened. We were so impressed with Josh's transformation that within a year we transferred his twin brother, Daniel.

Through the school we met many of the people involved in the Centre, including the authors of this book. No one ever pushed their beliefs on us or on the boys. It was simply plain for all to see that here was a group of extremely gentle, sincere, and dedicated people who really celebrated (as opposed to paying lip service to) the differences in each of us and wanted to do whatever they could to help us become all we could be, in mind, body, and spirit. In time, I took my first yoga classes at the Centre (advertised as Geezer Yoga). But it was not until I read some of the sections of this book, about the ancient traditions of Ayurveda, yoga, and spiritual practice, that I began to appreciate the many dimensions that make up life at the Salt Spring Centre. Even if these particular teachings are not your path, as they are not mine (Nancy practises Vipassana Buddhism and I am a follower of hers, but quite a long way behind), you cannot help but learn things that will enrich your own experience, if only peripherally. The traditions are presented in such a light and humorous way that, for me at least, they make understandable and relevant those teachings that have often been far from accessible.

Finally we get to the food, which is really my only credential for writing this foreword; I should probably have got to it sooner. I have always thought one of the great things about food is that it is a renewable pleasure. In moderation, we can all enjoy food two or three times a day without the slightest pang of guilt or feelings of self-indulgence, because we need it to go on living. Have a great meal and the next day (if not sooner) you are ready for another. And the variety is endless.

Food is also wonderfully flexible; depending on the food you choose, it can engender all manner of sensations: of well-being and pleasure, satisfaction, stimulation, and excitement—and, dare I say it, even of peace. This peaceful food is the kind they cook at the Salt Spring Centre, using many of the recipes in this book. Their meals are wholesome, satisfying, and calming, yet they have surprisingly complex flavours considering the simplicity of the ingredients.

The downside to pursuing a path to inner peace through eating is that, given the ephemeral nature of food, the peaceful feelings may not last very long. Besides, I have reluctantly come to the conclusion that in the search for lasting inner peace there is no substitute for dedication and application over a long period. This is too bad, because there is no doubt that cooking requires considerably less work than spiritual practice. The good news is that if you are in it for the long haul (and in the end who is not?), these recipes will sustain you through the hard times as well as the good times.

introduction

COME WITH US ON AN IMAGINARY JOURNEY to beautiful Salt Spring Island, the largest of British Columbia's Gulf Islands, just a short ferry ride from Vancouver.

Leaving for a well-deserved holiday can be hectic and you may feel tired or stressed, but we know you'll begin to unwind on your way to the island. Let's imagine it's a beautiful sunny day. You sit on the deck of the ferry, relax and enjoy the sunshine and the gentle breeze. We can picture your delight in the tranquility of the green islands, the ocean, and your first glimpse of Salt Spring.

The drive from the ferry dock to the Salt Spring Centre is short. In just a few minutes you turn into the tree-lined driveway. You receive a warm welcome and learn a bit about the Centre program you've come to attend. Dinner is at 6 p.m., so there is time to take a stroll through the garden or walk the woodland trail. You might like to sit and watch the deer that are grazing close by, apparently unconcerned by your arrival.

Just when you start to get hungry, someone steps out onto the back porch with a conch shell and raises it to her lips. A deep sound resonates through the valley. Because you're a first-time visitor and not sure about the conch's significance, someone explains that it's dinner time. Perfect timing!

Some of you may be new to vegetarian fare, and perhaps a bit apprehensive, but we know you'll enjoy the meal, and even come back for seconds. Our first book, *Salt Spring Island Cooking,* was born after years of writing recipes on scraps of paper in response to requests by guests. Of course, there are always more, and in this book we offer many new recipes as well as a lot more of what we do here at the Centre.

You may be curious about who we are and what the Salt Spring Centre is all about. We formed as a group in the Vancouver area 26 years ago to study and practise Ashtanga Yoga under the guidance of our teacher, Baba Hari Dass. After meeting in people's homes and rented halls for several years we began to dream about having a place of our own, a place in the country where people could visit and experience peace.

We made a number of exploratory trips before discovering the old heritage house on 70 acres of forest and meadow. We all knew right away that this was the place. The building was run down and in need of tender loving care, but it had character and charm, and we loved it. We renovated, built, plowed and planted, and still go on making changes.

Like the building, we continue to be transformed as we work together. Edges wear away and our goal of living in harmony becomes possible. We enjoy working and playing together, strengthening our yoga practice in our daily lives.

In the pages of this book, we welcome you to our home. We invite you to step into the kitchen to cook with us. Next, explore a bit of yoga philosophy and psychology, and then head off to your asana class. We invite you to discover health and fitness, Ayurveda style, and finally, in the spirit of play, we invite you to explore your inner self.

You may be more interested in one aspect than another. Take your time, go at your own speed and let your interest guide you as you journey through the pages.

We hope you enjoy your visit.

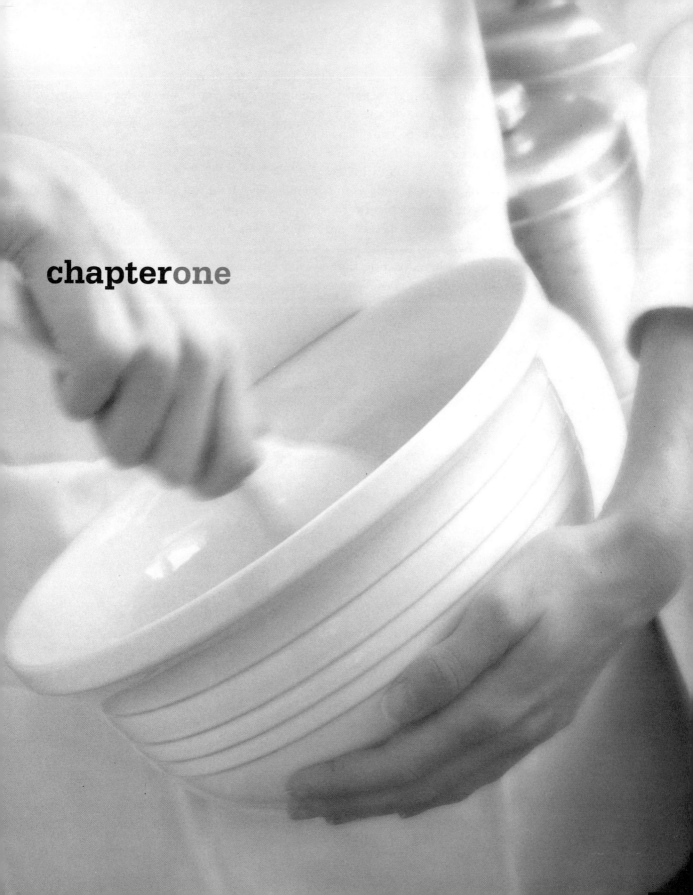

chapterone

from the kitchen:
more recipes from the salt spring centre

- Ingredients: What, How, and Why
- Soups
- Entrées
- World Food
- Veggies
- Salads and Dressing
- Sauces, Spreads, and Snacks
- Quick Breads and Muffins
- Desserts

WELCOME TO THE SALT SPRING CENTRE KITCHEN.

We're pleased to bring you more recipes from our kitchen, and to share with you what we've learned since we wrote *Salt Spring Island Cooking*.

The most important ingredient in any good kitchen is the joy of preparing and serving delicious, nourishing meals to family, friends, and guests.

Our Centre family includes people of many and varied talents, one of which is cooking. We frequently prepare delicious vegetarian meals for groups of 30 to 50 people, and up to 200 during our annual summer yoga retreats. Although it gets rather busy at times, it's amazing how smoothly it runs. This doesn't mean that we never have episodes of burnt rice or undercooked potatoes, but it does mean that we try to cultivate an attitude of peacefulness and unity so that we're not shaken by such situations. A good sense of humour helps, too.

Some of us have been here for many years, and some a few years or even a few months. Some are just passing through. All of us together make the Salt Spring Centre family. We welcome you to our kitchen on Salt Spring Island.

Ingredients:
What, How, and Why

Guests frequently ask us about the ingredients we use in the Centre's kitchen. If the ingredients are unfamiliar, they want to know how to use them. Visitors also ask regularly why we choose to use certain ingredients and avoid others. In these pages we shall attempt to answer these questions. As much as possible, categories are listed alphabetically.

Arrowroot Powder

Arrowroot powder or flour is an easily digested starch often used in baby foods and convalescent diets. It works well as a thickener, making a clear sauce.

Beans: Canned Versus Dried

It's always better to use dried rather than canned because dried beans have not been processed, nor do they have any additives. However, if you're preparing a dish that calls for beans and you don't have time to soak and cook them, it's okay to use canned. If you do, look for a brand that is organic and has the fewest possible additives.

Body Type

We've all noticed that people's bodies come in a variety of shapes and sizes—from extra small to extra large. What does that have to do with food? In the chapter on Ayurveda you'll find charts to determine your particular type, or dosha.

If you're trying to eat according to your constitution (your dosha), you can make adjustments to many recipes. One thing that's important to remember, however, is that the attitude with which you prepare and eat your food is as important as what you eat. Being anxious about what you eat can negate the benefits of even the healthiest food. Take your time, relax, and enjoy your meals.

TYPE OF BEAN	RATIO OF SOAKED BEANS TO WATER	COOK TIME (MIN)	YIELD (1 CUP DRY)
Aduki	1:4	40	3
Black Beans	1:1 1/2	40	2 1/3
Black Soybeans	1:2 1/2	90	2
Black Turtle	1:2	45	2 1/2
Brown Lentils	1:2	45	2 1/2
Garbanzos	1:3	40	2 1/2
Kidney	1:2	35	3
Limas (big)	1:2 1/2	40	2
Limas (small)	1:2 1/2	35	2
Mung Beans*	1:4	35	2 1/2
Navy Beans	1:2	30	2 1/2
Pintos	1:4	45	2 1/2
Red Lentils*	1:2	10	2
Soy Beans	1:4	2–4 hrs	2 1/2
Split Peas *	1:3	45	3

*do not require soaking

Note: Cooking times will also depend on the freshness of the beans. As well, whole mung beans take longer to cook than split mung.

Carob and Chocolate

Carob pods, which grow on trees, are picked and then ground into powder to be used in baking. If you need to avoid chocolate, carob is a good choice, but it's best not to think of carob as a chocolate substitute. Carob, also known as St. John's bread, has its own unique flavour. If you expect it to taste like chocolate you may be disappointed, but if you appreciate carob for itself you'll be able to enjoy its own delicious flavour. Unlike chocolate, carob is rich in vitamin B and minerals and is low in fats.

Dairy or Non-Dairy?

It's easier to be vegan these days because there are so many dairy alternatives available (at least on the West Coast). There are various soy and grain milks, many of which are made in more than one flavour. Depending on where you live, you may be able to find soy, rice, and oat milk, some made in regular and light (low-fat) versions. Although these products used to be the domain of natural food stores, many grocery stores now carry them as well.

You also have a choice in cheeses. There's a wide variety of dairy cheeses, mostly made from cow's milk, but some from goat's milk and sheep's milk. Most feta cheese in grocery stores is made from cow's milk, and is milder than that made from goat's or sheep's milk. Vegetarians need to read labels carefully to see what kind of rennet is used in the cheese-making process, since both animal and vegetable rennet are used. If you prefer to avoid dairy products, there are several soy or tofu cheeses on the market as well. You can even get soy parmesan in some places.

Butter is more difficult to substitute, although you can use oil instead of butter in many recipes. Substituting oil will alter the flavour somewhat because butter adds a sweetness that oil doesn't. Both butter and vegetable oil are preferable to margarine, which is a saturated fat.

Egg Replacer

Why egg replacer and not eggs? Because, at the Centre, we are strictly vegetarian, which includes the avoidance of eggs. However, if you eat eggs (and we suppose most people do), you can use eggs instead of egg replacer. One and a half teaspoons of egg replacer equals one egg.

Flours

Most flour used in baking is wheat of some kind. This is fine for most people, but many are allergic or sensitive to wheat. Many of the recipes in this book that contain wheat flour can be altered and made wheat-free.

Whole wheat flour works well for breads, while whole wheat pastry flour is lighter, and better for other baking. Unbleached white flour is lighter still.

Rye flour makes delicious bread, but it's heavy, and so is usually combined with wheat flour.

Spelt flour, which technically belongs to the wheat family, bakes much like whole wheat pastry flour. Many people who can't tolerate regular wheat flour are able to substitute spelt because it's lower in gluten. It's not suitable for people with celiac disease, however, because it does contain some gluten.

Kamut flour is considered by some to be the great-great-grandfather of grains. It's a variety of high protein wheat that has never been hybridized. Not only does it have a deliciously nutty flavour, but it also has a higher nutritional value than modern wheat. The gluten in kamut flour is said to be easier to digest than regular wheat gluten, so it can work as a wheat substitute for some people. Again, celiacs should avoid it because it does contain gluten.

Brown rice flour contains no gluten, so is usually combined with wheat flour to keep the dough from crumbling. It can be used alone when combined with soaked flaxseed; it will hold together beautifully when baked. For every cup of brown rice flour, use 2 tablespoons of ground flax seed soaked for 15 minutes in 2 tablespoons cup of hot water. Add it to the wet ingredients in the recipe.

Fennel

Chewing a handful of fennel seeds after a meal will help your digestion and sweeten your breath at the same time.

Flaxseed

Flaxseed is somewhat of a wonder food, being the richest food source of alpha-linolenic acid, a type of omega-3 fat that helps prevent heart attacks by reducing potentially deadly blood clots and abnormal heart rhythms. It's high in fibre, and is also a rich plant source of lignins, a type of phyto estrogen, which may reduce the risk of cancer. Although broccoli is considered a high source of antioxidants, flaxseed has 75 times more. It's also high in vitamins and minerals, especially potassium. Grind it up to eat it; otherwise, it will pass through the digestive tract undigested.

Ginger

Fresh ginger root has a very different flavour from powdered ginger. Unless otherwise specified, recipes calling for ginger refer to fresh ginger root.

Grains

Grains require cooking before they're used in a recipe. Bulgar is an exception, needing only to be soaked in boiling water. Here's a preparation chart, much like that for beans.

TYPE OF GRAIN	GRAIN/ WATER RATIO	COOK TIME (MIN)	YIELD (CUPS)
Barley	1:2 1/2	60	3
Basmati Rice	1:1/2	20	2
Brown Rice	1: 2	50	2
Buckwheat	1:1 3/4	30	2
Bulgur	1:2	15	2 1/2
Cornmeal	1:4	30	3 1/2
Cracked Wheat	1:3	20	2 1/2
Millet	1:2	40	3 1/2
Quinoa*	1:1 1/2 or 2	15	3
Wheat Berries	1:5	90	3

*Quinoa must be rinsed. See Daya's Quinoa Salad (page 64) for instructions.

Herbs

Most of us buy dried herbs and spices, either in containers or in bulk. There are times, though, when some fresh herbs are available in stores—or better yet, from your own garden. Many are easy to grow on the windowsill in your kitchen.

What's good about them? Organic farmers use methods that neither deplete the soil nor harm environmental systems or farm workers. Yes, but are organic foods healthier than commercial foods? Some commercial products are nutritionally depleted, but even when you don't know the difference in nutrition, the lack of synthetic pesticidal residues on organically grown produce definitely makes for a safer product.

Rice

Two kinds of rice are used in the recipes in this book—brown rice and basmati rice. Brown rice comes in long or short grain, while basmati, an Indian rice, comes in both brown and white. Brown rice, whether long or short grain, takes about 50 minutes to cook once it's brought to a boil. Brown basmati takes almost as long, while white basmati cooks in 15 to 20 minutes after it's brought to a boil. Cover the pot when cooking rice. There is more nutritional value in brown rice, but some people find basmati easier to digest. Use whichever you prefer.

Seaweed

There are many varieties of seaweed available, usually at natural food stores or Japanese food stores. The one most familiar to North Americans is nori, which is used to wrap sushi. All seaweeds are very high in minerals.

Shitake Mushrooms

Shitake mushrooms are sometimes available fresh in grocery stores. If you can't find them, try a store that sells Asian foods. You can also buy dried shitake and dried Chinese mushrooms in Japanese or Chinese food stores. These need to be reconstituted by soaking them in water.

Sweeteners

Another question that often arises is "Why do you bake with sugar now instead of honey?" It's true that in our first book we baked with honey, and that we've now switched to sugar (or maple syrup). The reason is that we've learned more about Ayurveda, which says that heating honey destroys its beneficial properties and turns it into a harmful substance.

To most people, sugar means white sugar. However, there are other choices. We usually use turbinado sugar, which is one of several organic raw sugars. Others are Sucanat and demerara. Be aware that demerara-style is not the same as raw demerara sugar, which is an unrefined dark-brown sugar. Ordinary brown sugar, which can be bought in any grocery store, is refined beet or cane sugar with molasses added for colouring.

Maple syrup is made from the sap of the sugar maple tree. It takes 35 gallons of sap to make one gallon of syrup. Yes, it's expensive, but it's also delicious.

When we refer to molasses in a recipe, we're talking about blackstrap molasses, which is a dark molasses with a fairly strong flavour. It's what's left over when sugar is processed, and contains all the minerals leached out of sugar during refining.

Unpasteurized honey contains many minerals, enzymes, and some B vitamins. If you store honey in a warm, dry place, it will last for years. It's the world's oldest sweetener, and is sweeter than sugar. Just don't heat it.

Ayurveda recommends the following sweeteners for different body/mind types: Vatta—raw sugar; Pitta—brown sugar;

Kapha—honey. The main thing to remember is that excess carbohydrates, including sugars, are not healthy for any body/mind type. However, in moderation, they can be part of a balanced diet.

Tahini

Tahini is a paste made of ground sesame seeds (much like a nut butter), and is used widely in the Middle East. It's available at most natural food stores. Because it becomes rancid quickly, it must be kept refrigerated.

Tamari and Bragg's

Both tamari and Bragg's All Purpose Seasoning (which we usually refer to as Bragg's) are made from fermented soybeans. Neither has any additives, and both are superior in flavour to regular store-bought soy sauce. Try both tamari and Bragg's, and see which you prefer—and they're also good in combination. If you have a wheat allergy, be aware that some brands of tamari contain wheat, so read labels carefully. Tamari and Bragg's may be available at your local grocery store. If not, try a natural food store (or an Asian food store for tamari).

Tofu

Tofu, made from soybeans, is a complete protein with all eight essential amino acids. It's low in calories, fats, and carbohydrates, and has no cholesterol. Tofu is also very versatile. There are several varieties available, ranging from firm to very soft. We generally use a fairly firm tofu, but prefer the softer silken tofu in dessert recipes. Because it's packaged in foil-lined boxes, silken tofu has a long shelf life. Regular tofu should be stored in water, and kept refrigerated.

Changing the water every day keeps it fresh for a longer period of time.

Vegetarian Diet

For many of our guests, eating only vegetarian food is a new experience, and they're often delightfully surprised by how much they enjoy the food. It was their frequent requests for recipes that prompted us to write our first book, *Salt Spring Island Cooking*. Many people have moved toward vegetarian diets for health reasons, a valid (and probably the most common) reason for becoming vegetarian. Another reason for being vegetarian is the desire to live a lifestyle that creates as little harm to living creatures as possible.

Vinegar

The word *vinegar* is derived from the French *vin aigre,* or sour wine. It is made by bacterial activity that converts fermented liquids into a weak solution of acetic acid, which makes the vinegar sour. There are several kinds from which to choose.

Balsamic vinegar, which comes from Italy, is made from white Trebbiano grape juice. It gets its dark colour and pungent sweetness from aging in barrels.

Cider vinegar, which is made from fermented apple cider, has a mild, fruity flavour.

Herb vinegars are made by steeping fresh herbs such as dill or tarragon in vinegar.

Malt vinegar is made from malted barley.

Rice vinegar, made from fermented rice, is widely used in Japanese and Chinese cooking.

Wine vinegar is made from either red or white wine.

Yeast (Engevita and Nutritional)

Neither engevita nor nutritional yeast is a leavening yeast, like that used in bread making. Rather, they serve as a condiment and ingredient in some recipes. Engevita and nutritional yeast are similar in their nutritional benefits, both of them containing B vitamins, but many people prefer the almost nutty flavour of engevita yeast, and sprinkle it generously on grains, vegetables, and soups.

ali baba's soup

SERVES 4–6

This is a mild and delicately flavoured soup, with sesame tahini being Ali Baba's secret ingredient.

2 cups (480 mL) chopped leeks

4 Tbsp (60 mL) olive oil

2 cups (480 mL) chopped carrots

1 1/2 cups (360 mL) chopped celery

4 cups (960 mL) sliced mushrooms

2–4 Tbsp (30–60 mL) grated or
minced ginger

1 cup (240 mL) tahini

4 cups (960 mL) water

4 Tbsp (60 mL) tamari

1/2–1 tsp (2–5 mL) salt

2–2 1/2 cups (480–600 mL) cubed
tofu

Pinch cayenne

1. Sauté the leeks in olive oil until they begin to soften. Add the carrots and celery and sauté a bit longer before adding the mushrooms and ginger. Sauté all together for 3 or 4 minutes.

2. In a blender, blend the tahini with the water.

3. Add the rest of the ingredients to the pot. Bring to a boil, then turn the heat down to simmer. Cover and cook for half an hour or until the vegetables are soft and the flavour is released into the broth. Add a bit more water if you prefer a thinner soup. (If you do add water, simmer for a few more minutes before serving.)

alicia's almond-coconut vegetable soup

SERVES 4–6

This unusual soup was created by Alicia, our youngest cook and a true artist in the kitchen. The combination of root vegetables, coconut milk, and almond butter is richly delicious.

1. Bring the water to a boil in a large saucepan, and add the potatoes and yams. Cover the pot, reduce the heat, and cook for 15–20 minutes, or until the vegetables are soft. Sauté the leeks and spices in olive oil over medium-high heat for 2–3 minutes, then add them to the pot.

2. In a blender, blend the almond butter and coconut milk. Stir the mixture into the soup.

3. Add the kale last. Cover the pot and let it cook on low heat for approximately 10–15 minutes. When the kale is soft, the soup is done.

4 cups (960 mL) water

3 cups (720 mL) cubed potatoes, peeled or scrubbed

3 cups (720 mL) cubed yams, peeled or scrubbed

4 Tbsp (60 mL) olive oil

1 cup (240 mL) chopped leeks

1/2–1 tsp (2–5 mL) rosemary

1/2–1 tsp (2–5 mL) salt

1/2 tsp (2 mL) pepper

1/2 cup (120 mL) almond butter

13.5-oz tin (400 mL) coconut milk

3 cups (720 mL) chopped kale

ALICIA HAS BEEN COMING TO YOGA RETREATS at the Salt Spring Centre since she was a little girl. At about age 10 she started helping in the Centre's kitchen. By age 15 she was coming regularly to help cook at Women's Weekends. Her specialty became presentation, making sure that everything served was exquisitely decorated with herbs and flowers. Now, at the ripe old age of 17, she's developed a number of recipes of her own. One day she'll undoubtedly put together her own cookbook.

borscht

SERVES 8–10

Although this is similar to other borscht recipes, Sharada, one of the main cooks at the Centre, makes hers extra special by adding more spices, lemon, and sugar.

4 cups (960 mL) coarsely grated
  raw beets

2 cups (480 mL) coarsely grated
  raw potatoes

2 cups (480 mL) chopped leeks

3 bay leaves, tied in cheesecloth

8 cups (1.92 L) water

1–2 tsp (5–10 mL) salt

1/2 tsp (2 mL) pepper

1 1/2 Tbsp (22 mL) dillweed

1/2–3/4 cup (120–180 mL) turbinado
  sugar

1/2–3/4 cup (120–180 mL) fresh
  lemon juice

1. Place the grated beets and potatoes, chopped leeks, and bay leaves in a saucepan with the water, and bring the water to a boil. Then cover, reduce the heat, and simmer for 10–15 minutes.

2. Add the rest of the ingredients. Cover and simmer for at least half an hour.

3. Remove the bay leaves.

4. Serve the borscht with a dollop of yogurt or sour cream.

coconut-ginger yam soup

SERVES 8–10

This soup was inspired by Southeast Asian cuisine. Ginger and coconut milk impart a spicy sweetness.

1. Boil the water in a soup pot and place the yams, carrots, and leeks in the pot with the water. Bring to a boil again, then cover and simmer for 15–20 minutes or until the vegetables are soft.
2. Add the ginger, spices, and coconut milk (or coconut milk and water if you prefer the soup less rich).
3. Blend the soup in a blender, then return it to the pot. Cover and simmer for another half an hour.

6 cups (1.54 L) cubed yams

2 cups (480 mL) chopped carrots

1 cup (240 mL) chopped leeks

7 cups (1.68 L) water

1 Tbsp (15 mL) finely grated ginger

1 tsp (5 mL) garam masala

1 tsp (5 mL) cinnamon

1 tsp (5 mL) salt

Pinch of cayenne

2 13.5-oz tins (800 mL) coconut milk or 13.5-oz tin (400 mL) coconut milk and 1 2/3 cups (400 mL) water

TIPS   COCONUT MILK

• If you prefer a richer, sweeter soup, use two tins of coconut milk instead of the combination of coconut milk and water.

creamy mushroom soup

A gnome's favourite—especially vegan gnomes (though it doesn't have to be vegan). To make this soup vegan, simply use vegetable oil instead of ghee (clarified butter, page 41) and soymilk instead of milk.

2 cups (480 mL) chopped leeks

2 Tbsp (30 mL) vegetable oil
or ghee (page 41)

5 cups (1.2 L) finely chopped
mushrooms

3 Tbsp (45 mL) flour

5 cups (1.2 L) milk or soymilk

1 tsp (5 mL) salt

1/2 tsp (2 mL) pepper

2 tsp (10 mL) dillweed

2 tsp (10 mL) basil

1/2 cup (120 mL) finely minced
parsley

1. Sauté the leeks in ghee (or oil) over medium heat in a saucepan. Add the mushrooms, and cook until they're soft.

2. Sprinkle the flour over the mushrooms and leeks and stir it in, making sure there are no lumps.

3. Add the milk (or soymilk), salt and pepper, and herbs. Bring the soup to a boil, then cover and turn the heat down to low. Simmer for half an hour.

4. Serve sprinkled with parmesan (regular or soy).

creamy tomato basil soup

SERVES 4-6

If you're trying to lose weight, don't eat this soup—turn the page!
Delicious—reminiscent of old Italy and warm Mediterranean winds.

1. Boil the water in a pot, add the tomatoes, and boil them for 5–10 minutes until the peels split. Remove from the water and peel, core, and chop them.
2. In a saucepan, sauté the leeks in olive oil.
3. Add the chopped tomatoes, 4 cups water, salt and pepper, and basil to the leeks.
4. Cover the pot and simmer 1–1 1/2 hours. Ten minutes before serving, stir in the cream.

16 Roma tomatoes
2 cups (480 mL) chopped leeks
2 Tbsp (30 mL) olive oil
4 cups (960 mL) water
2 tsp (10 mL) salt
1/2 tsp (2 mL) pepper
2 Tbsp (30 mL) dry basil or
  3/4–1 cup (180–240 mL)
  fresh basil, minced
1/2 cup (120 mL) whipping cream

THIS RECIPE IS FROM DONNA, who spends quite a lot of time at the Salt Spring Centre. She has two children in the school, and as a member of the Centre's Health Collective, gives health treatments to guests. Donna also happens to be a great cook.

golden squash soup

SERVES 4–6

Beautiful to behold and a delight to eat. Cinderella would probably have made this soup on that fateful night when her carriage turned back into a butternut squash.

5 1/2–6 lb (2.75–3 kg) butternut
squash (or another rich winter
squash like Hubbard)
6 cups (1.54 L) water
2 cups (480 mL) chopped leeks
1/3 cup (80 mL) butter or
ghee (page 41) or vegetable oil
1 tsp (5 mL) salt
1 Tbsp (15 mL) tamari
Pinch cayenne

1. Cut the squash in half lengthwise. Place it face down in a baking pan with a bit of water, and bake it at 400°F (205°C) for about half an hour—until the squash is soft.

2. When it's done, scoop the squash flesh from the peel and mash it. It should give you about 6 cups (1.54 L) of mashed squash.

3. Blend the squash pulp with water in a blender. It's easiest if you do it in 3 batches, with 2 cups (480 mL) squash to 2 cups water.

4. Pour the squash and water mixture into a saucepan and bring to a boil. Then cover it, turn the heat down, and let it simmer while you prepare the leeks.

5. In a frying pan, sauté the leeks in butter or ghee until the leeks are soft and add them to the soup.

6. Add the salt, tamari, and cayenne. Cover and simmer for 20 minutes or more before serving.

minestrone

A great soup for wintry evenings—full, robust, and comforting.

1. Soak the beans overnight, then cook in 2 cups boiling water until soft. (Or skip this step and use 2 cups [480 mL] canned kidney beans.)
2. Cook the pasta and set it aside.
3. Sauté the vegetables in olive oil until soft.
4. Place all ingredients except the parmesan, parsley, and pasta into a large pot. Bring to a boil, then cover and simmer for 40 minutes or until the flavours of the vegetables are released.
5. Add the remaining ingredients before serving.

2/3 cup (160 mL) dried kidney beans
1/2 cup (120 mL) uncooked pasta
4 1/2 cups (1.08 L) chopped leeks
2 cups (480 mL) chopped celery
3 cups (720 mL) chopped carrots
3 cups (720 mL) chopped zucchini
1 cup (240 mL) grated red cabbage
1 1/2 tsp (7 mL) salt
1 tsp (5 mL) black pepper
3 Tbsp (45 mL) oregano
1/4 cup (60 mL) olive oil
2 Tbsp (30 mL) basil
8 cups (1.92 L) water
2 cups (480 mL) canned crushed tomatoes
2 cups (480 mL) chopped fresh tomatoes
1/2–3/4 cup (120–180 mL) parmesan cheese
1 cup (240 mL) minced parsley

miso soup

SERVES 6–8

A deliciously warming and soothing soup. Miso is made from fermented soybeans. In addition to tasting good, it's good for digestion.

11 cups (2.16 L) **water**

3–4 Tbsp (180–240 mL) grated fresh ginger

3 cups (720 mL) **thinly** sliced carrots

2 cups (480 mL) **thinly** sliced leeks

2 cups (480 mL) **chopped** kale

3 cups (720 mL) **sliced, fresh shitake mushrooms**

1 cup (240 mL) **cubed** tofu

1/4–1/2 cup (60–120 mL) nori seaweed, cut **into** strips (optional)

2/3 cup (160 mL) **brown** rice miso

1. In a saucepan, bring the water and ginger to a boil. Cover and simmer for 15–20 minutes.

2. Add the vegetables and tofu. Cover and cook until the vegetables are soft and the flavour is released into the broth. Remove from heat and allow to cool slightly.

3. Ladle out one cup of the broth and place it in a bowl. Mix the miso into the broth, then return the mixture to the soup. Add the seaweed and serve.

TIPS MISO

• Reheating the soup once the miso is added destroys the micro-organisms and enzymes that aid digestion.

plato's greek lentil soup

It's a little-known fact that Plato actually invented this soup while writing *The Republic,* which is why you'll find it so balanced.

1. Pick over the lentils, removing any tiny twigs or stones.

2. Rinse the lentils and put them in a pot with the water, 1/2 cup olive oil, and bay leaves. Add the salt, pepper, and oregano.

3. Sauté the leeks and carrots in the 5 tablespoons of olive oil for 3 or 4 minutes, then add them to the soup.

4. Add the tomato paste and vinegar. Cover and simmer. The lentils will get mushy. Cook for at least half an hour or until the flavours are well blended.

5. Remove the bay leaves before serving.

3 cups (720 mL) dried red lentils

12 cups (2.9 L) water

1/2 cup (120 mL) olive oil

6 large bay leaves, tied in cheese cloth

1–2 tsp (5–10 mL) salt

1/2 tsp (2 mL) pepper

3 Tbsp (45 mL) oregano

3 cups (720 mL) chopped leeks

2 cups (480 mL) chopped carrots

5 Tbsp (75 mL) olive oil

1/3 cup (80 mL) tomato paste

1 Tbsp (15 mL) apple cider vinegar

potato-leek soup

SERVES 8

Simple but elegant. A good starter for any meal.

4 cups (960 mL) chopped leeks

5 Tbsp (75 mL) olive oil

6 cups (1.54 L) cubed potatoes,
  peeled or scrubbed

7 cups (1.68 L) water

4 bay leaves, tied in cheesecloth

6 Tbsp (90 mL) tamari

1 1/2 tsp (7 mL) salt

1/2 tsp (2 mL) pepper

1 cup (240 mL) minced fresh parsley

3 Tbsp (45 mL) ghee (page 41)
  (optional)

1. Sauté the leeks in olive oil. Add the potatoes and sauté briefly.

2. Add the water, bay leaves, and the rest of the ingredients. Cover and bring to a boil. Then turn down the heat and let the soup simmer at least half an hour or until the flavours are well blended.

3. If you prefer a smoother soup, mix it in a blender before serving. Remove the bay leaves first.

4. Serve sprinkled with parmesan cheese.

almond-rice casserole

SERVES 6

A complete meal in a dish. The vegetables in the filling can be varied to suit your taste.

Rice Layer:
1. In a frying pan, sauté the peppers and leeks in the olive oil until they're soft.
2. Add the peppers and leeks to the cooked rice in a large bowl. Toss in the rest of the ingredients, except the almonds.
3. Press half the mixture into an oiled casserole dish. Reserve the other half for the top layer.

Filling:
1. Sprinkle salt on the peeled and chopped eggplant and set it aside for about 15 minutes, then rinse.
2. Sauté the eggplant, corn, leeks, broccoli, herbs, and spices in olive oil and tamari until the vegetables start to soften, but are still firm (al dente).
3. Spread the filling over the rice in the casserole dish.
4. For the top layer, spread the other half of the rice mixture over the filling and press it down. Sprinkle the almonds on top and bake at 325°F (165°C) for 20 to 25 minutes, until the top is browned.

Rice layer:
7 cups (1.68 L) cooked basmati rice
1 cup (240 mL) chopped peppers
2 1/2 cups (600 mL) chopped leeks
2 Tbsp (30 mL) olive oil
1 cup (240 mL) pitted and chopped
   Greek olives
2 Tbsp (30 mL) parsley flakes
1 Tbsp (15 mL) oregano
1 Tbsp (15 mL) basil
1/2 tsp (2 mL) salt
1/2 tsp (2 mL) pepper
2 cups (480 mL) crushed almonds

Filling:
5 cups (1.2 L) peeled and chopped
   eggplant
Salt
2 cups (480 mL) frozen corn
2 1/3 cups (560 mL) chopped leeks
3 cups (720 mL) broccoli
2 Tbsp (30 mL) basil
3 Tbsp (45 mL) oregano
1 tsp (5 mL) salt
1/2 tsp (2 mL) pepper
1/4 cup (60 mL) olive oil
1/4 cup (60 mL) tamari

breaded and baked tofu

SERVES 8–10

B&B tofu makes a quick-to-prepare protein meal that everyone enjoys. While it's baking, prepare your vegetable and rice and salad. If time is short, the tofu can be pan fried instead of baked.

Breading:
1/2 cup (120 mL) cornmeal
3/4 cup (180 mL) engevita yeast
3/4 cup (180 mL) sesame seeds
1 Tbsp (15 mL) dillweed
2 tsp (7–10 mL) basil
Pinch cayenne

2 lb (1 kg) tofu
1/2 cup (120 mL) tamari

1. Combine the cornmeal, yeast, sesame seeds, herbs, and cayenne to make the breading mixture.
2. Set out two bowls, one for tamari and one for the breading mixture.
3. Slice the tofu into 1/4 to 1/2 inch (1/2 to 1 cm) slices (your preference).
4. Dip each piece of tofu first into the tamari, and then into the breading mixture, making sure it's well coated.
5. Place the tofu slices on an oiled baking tray and bake at 375°F (190°C) 35 to 45 minutes, depending on how crispy you like them.

TIPS   BREADING

• Any leftover breading mixture can be refrigerated or frozen for next time.

donna's black bean and rice pie

SERVES 6–8

Donna, a gifted healer, both in the massage room and in the kitchen, brings us this delicately flavoured, nourishing dish—a feast for the eyes as well as for the palate. It holds its shape well when cut, which makes it great for lunches.

Crust
1. In a food processor, blend the flour, salt, and butter until the mixture resembles small pebbles.
2. While the food processor is still going, slowly add the milk until the mixture forms a ball.
3. Chill the dough for half an hour before using. When chilled, roll out the dough and press it into a pie plate. Oil or butter the plate first to make it easier to serve.

Filling
1. In a frying pan, sauté the leeks in oil until they're golden.
2. In a large bowl, combine the leeks with all the other ingredients and pour into the piecrust.
3. Bake at 400°F (205°C) for 10 minutes, then reduce the heat to 375°F (190°C) and bake another 45 minutes to 1 hour—until the crust is golden and the filling has set.

Crust:
1 cup (240 mL) flour (whole wheat pasty or spelt)
1/2 tsp (2 mL) salt
4 Tbsp (60 mL) butter
5–6 Tbsp (75–90 mL) milk or soymilk

Filling:
2 Tbsp (30 mL) olive or vegetable oil
2 cups (480 mL) chopped leeks
1 cup (240 mL) cooked black beans
2 cups (480 mL) cooked basmati rice
1 cup (240 mL) milk or soymilk
1 Tbsp (15 mL) egg replacer mixed with 2 Tbsp (30 mL) of water
1/2 tsp (2 mL) salt
2 tsp (10 mL) tarragon
3/4 cup (180 mL) grated cheese (dairy or soy)

ginger-chili stir fry

SERVES 4–6

Short for time? This cooks up quickly and easily, and wakes up your taste buds at the same time! Great over rice.

4 Tbsp (60 mL) vegetable oil

2 cups (480 mL) cubed tofu

5 Tbsp (75 mL) tamari

2 cups (480 mL) thinly sliced leeks (rounds)

3 Tbsp (45 mL) grated ginger

3/4 cup (180 mL) water

5 cups (1.2 L) broccoli pieces

1 Tbsp (15 mL) chili powder

3 Tbsp (45 mL) turbinado sugar

1. Heat the oil in a wok or frying pan over quite high heat.
2. Add the tofu and stir-fry briefly.
3. Add 2 tablespoons (30 mL) tamari, stirring to brown all the edges of the tofu.
4. Add the leeks and ginger and 3 to 4 tablespoons (45 to 60 mL) of water. Keep stirring.
5. Add the broccoli and 1/2 cup (120 mL) of water, continuing to stir.
6. Add the chili powder, sugar, and 3 tablespoons (45 mL) tamari. Mix everything in, then cover the pan and turn the heat down a bit. Cook until the broccoli is soft, but still bright green. (If you want more sauce, add another 1/4 to 1/2 cup [60 to 120 mL] of water before you put the cover on.)

martha's nut loaf

A protein-rich main course, delicious on its own or served with Tahini-Ginger Sauce (page 87) or Eggplant Relish (page 85).

1. Mix the rice and nuts together in a mixing bowl.
2. Sauté the leeks in olive oil, and add them to the rice and nut mixture.
3. Add the remaining ingredients and mix well.
4. Press the mixture into an oiled baking pan, and bake at 350°F (180°C) for 45 to 50 minutes.

2 cups (480 mL) ground almonds
   and/or cashews
2 cups (480 mL) cooked brown rice
4 Tbsp (60 mL) olive oil
2 cups (480 mL) chopped leeks
1 1/2 cups (360 mL) chopped celery
1 1/2 cups (360 mL) grated carrots
1/2 cup (120 mL) pitted and
   chopped Greek olives
1 tsp (5 mL) salt
1/2 tsp (2 mL) pepper
2 Tbsp (30 mL) basil
2 Tbsp (30 mL) dillweed
1 1/2 cups (360 mL) grated dairy or
   tofu cheese
1/3 cup (80 mL) flour
1/3 cup (80 mL) water

WE HADN'T SEEN MARTHA SINCE she moved to Toronto to become a computer expert 20 years ago, and she called to say she was on Salt Spring. Could she come and visit? Of course! We were testing recipes, and she was drawn right in. This is her contribution.

nayana's mediterranean tofu quiche

SERVES 6–8

So tasty, so pretty, that anyone who doesn't like tofu will be immediately won over by this rich and unusual pie. Magnifico!

Crust

1. Mix the sesame seeds, flour, and salt in a food processor. Add the parsley, then the oil.
2. Add the water last. Mix only until the dough holds together. Roll out the dough and fit it into a greased pie plate.

Crust:

1 cup (240 mL) toasted, ground
    sesame seeds

2 cups (480 mL) flour (whole wheat
    pastry or spelt)

1/2 cup (120 mL) minced fresh
    parsley

1/2 tsp (2 mL) salt

1/2 cup (120 mL) vegetable oil

3/4 cup (180 mL) cold water

Filling:

4 Tbsp (60 mL) olive oil

2 cups (480 mL) chopped leeks

4 cups (960 mL) chopped zucchini

1–1 1/2 cups (240–360 mL) chopped
   peppers (red, green, or yellow)

2 cups (480 mL) chopped fresh
   tomatoes

1/2 cup (120 mL) pitted and
   chopped Greek olives

1 cup (240 mL) chopped artichoke
   hearts

4 Tbsp (60 mL) flour

1/2 tsp (2 mL) salt

1/2 tsp (2 mL) pepper

3 Tbsp (45 mL) oregano

2 Tbsp (30 mL) basil

2–2 1/2 cups (480–600 mL)
   blended tofu

2 cups (480 mL) grated or
   crumbled feta

Filling

1. Sauté the leeks in oil. Add the zucchini, peppers, tomatoes, olives, and artichokes. Cover and cook for 10 to 15 minutes, or until the vegetables are soft.

2. Stir in the flour. Add the spices and mix them in.

3. Mix in the tofu.

4. Turn the heat off and mix in half of the feta.

5. Place the mixture into the pie shell, and sprinkle the remaining feta over the top.

6. Bake at 350°F (180°C) for 40 to 45 minutes.

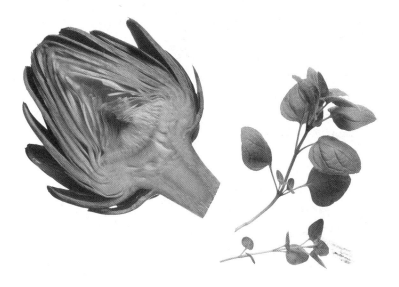

nayana's
curried tofu quiche

SERVES 6-8

A cleverly disguised tofu quiche—this time an East Indian curry. As long as you have 6 cups (1.54 mL) raw vegetables for the filling, you can change the ratio to whatever you prefer.

Crust:

1 cup (240 mL) toasted, ground
  sesame seeds

2 cups (480 mL) flour (whole wheat
  pastry or spelt)

1/2 tsp (2 mL) salt

1/2 cup (120 mL) vegetable oil

3/4 cup (180 mL) cold water

Filling:

5 Tbsp (75 mL) vegetable oil

2 cups (480 mL) chopped leeks

2-3 Tbsp (30–45 mL) grated ginger

2 tsp (10 mL) ground coriander

1 Tbsp (15 mL) ground cumin

2 tsp (10 mL) turmeric

1 Tbsp (15 mL) garam masala

1 Tbsp (15 mL) chili powder

1/2 tsp (2 mL) salt

4 cups (960 mL) cauliflower pieces

1 cup (240 mL) cubed potatoes

1 cup (240 mL) peas

1–1 1/2 cups (240–360 mL) water

2–2 1/2 cups (480–600 mL)
  blended tofu

Crust

1. Mix the ground sesame seeds, flour, and salt in a food processor, then add the oil.
2. Add the water last. Mix only until the dough holds together. Roll out the dough and fit it into a greased pie plate.

Filling

1. Sauté the leeks and ginger in the oil.
2. Add the spices and mix them in. Sauté briefly.
3. Add the vegetables and the water. Cover the pan and simmer until the vegetables are soft.
4. Mix the tofu in with the vegetables.
5. Place the mixture in the pie shell and bake at 350°F (180°C) for 40 to 45 minutes.

sid's tofu scramble

A spicy alternative to eggs—great with buttered rye or sourdough rye toast or rolled in a tortilla. Sid, our local jalapeno aficionado, swears this recipe came down from the ancient Aztecs—revealed to him in a vision.

1. In a wok or large frying pan, sauté the leeks and green peppers in olive oil over medium-high heat.
2. Add the rest of the ingredients, stirring regularly until the tomatoes are cooked in.

2 Tbsp (30 mL) olive oil
1 cup (240 mL) chopped leeks
2 cups (480 mL) chopped green peppers
6 cups (1.54 L) crumbled tofu
2 cups (480 mL) chopped tomatoes
5 Tbsp (75 mL) tamari
4 Tbsp (60 mL) balsamic vinegar
1 Tbsp (15 mL) turmeric
1 Tbsp (15 mL) turbinado sugar
2 finely minced pickled jalapeno peppers
1/4 cup (60 mL) pitted and chopped Greek olives (optional)

TIPS   JALAPENOS

• You can adjust the spiciness by using fewer (or more) jalapenos.

sid's wild tofu surprise

SERVES 6–8

Bugs Bunny fans may remember the Wild Turkey Surprise that Bugs prepared for the Tasmanian Devil. This is the nourishing vegetarian version.

2 Tbsp (30 mL) olive oil

1/2 cup (120 mL) chopped leeks

3–3 1/2 cups (720–840 mL) cubed
  tofu (about 1 lb)

1 cup (240 mL) water

Pinch chili flakes (optional)

3 rounded Tbsp (45 mL) chili
  powder (or less for a milder
  version)

2 Tbsp (30 mL) tamari

2 cups (480 mL) cubed zucchini or
  chopped green beans

3 cups (720 mL) peppers (red,
  yellow, or green), cut into strips

2 cups (480 mL) sliced mushrooms

2 cups (480 mL) chopped tomatoes

1 tsp (5 mL) Dijon mustard

1 1/2 tsp (7 mL) balsamic vinegar

4 rounded Tbsp (60 mL) turbinado
  sugar

Pinch salt

Pinch pepper

Roasted sesame oil

1. Heat the oil in a wok or a large frying pan over high heat.
2. When the oil is hot, add the leeks, and stir-fry them until they're lightly browned.
3. Add the tofu and 1/4 cup (60 mL) of water.
4. When the tofu begins to brown, turn the heat down to medium.
5. Add the chili flakes and chili powder. Stir until all the tofu cubes are well coated.
6. Add the tamari, and continue stirring for 2 to 3 minutes.
7. Add 1/3 cup (80 mL) of water and the zucchini (or beans) and peppers. Cook for 3 to 4 minutes, stirring regularly.
8. Add the mushrooms and tomatoes, and cook them until soft. Keep stirring.
9. Add the mustard, balsamic vinegar, sugar, salt, pepper, and the rest of the water. Reduce the heat to medium-low and allow to simmer for another 4 to 5 minutes.
10. Serve over rice and drizzle with roasted sesame oil before serving.

winter vegetable stew

SERVES 6–8

A hearty, down-to-earth meal in a bowl. Best eaten on a cold day with thick slices of bread.

1. In a large pot, sauté the leeks in oil until they become soft.

2. Add the potatoes, yams, carrots, and water. Cover the pot and cook the vegetables for 15 to 20 minutes or until they begin to get soft.

3. Add all the remaining ingredients except the flour, and mix everything together. Cover and cook over medium-low heat for 15 to 20 minutes.

4. Sprinkle the flour over the top of the vegetables and mix it in, making sure there are no lumps of flour left.

5. Cover and simmer for half an hour or until the vegetables are soft and the flavours are blended.

5 Tbsp (75 mL) olive oil

3 cups (720 mL) chopped leeks

3 cups (720 mL) cubed potatoes, scrubbed or peeled

2 cups (480 mL) cubed yams, scrubbed or peeled

2 cups (480 mL) chopped carrots

3 cups (720 mL) water

2 cups (480 mL) frozen peas

1 tsp (5 mL) salt

1/2 tsp (2 mL) pepper

1 Tbsp (15 mL) basil

1 Tbsp (15 mL) dillweed

1 cup (240 mL) fresh minced parsley

3 Tbsp (45 mL) tamari

1 tsp (5 mL) Dijon mustard

1/4 cup (60 mL) flour

TIPS   VEGGIE PIE

- This stew can also be made into a veggie pie by spooning the stew into a prepared pie shell.
- You can add a top pie crust or sprinkle the top with cheese (cheddar, mozzarella, parmesan, soy cheese—the choice is yours).
- Then bake the pie for 30 to 40 minutes at 350°F (180°C).

harvest stuffed zucchini

SERVES 8–12

A dressed-up, elegant use for the big zucchini that got away—or her smaller relatives.

1 cup (240 mL) cooked basmati rice

3 medium zucchinis (or 1 large one)

1 cup (240 mL) chopped leeks

3 Tbsp (45 mL) olive oil

1/2 cup (120 mL) minced fresh dillweed (or 3 Tbsp [45 mL] dry, but
   use fresh if you can get it)

2 Tbsp (30 mL) basil

1 Tbsp (15 mL) oregano

1/2 tsp (2 mL) salt

1/2 tsp (2 mL) pepper

1/2 cup (120 mL) chopped almonds

1/2 cup (120 mL) crushed canned
   tomatoes

2 Tbsp (30 mL) tamari

1 1/2 cups (360 mL) grated cheese

(of your preference—cheddar,
   mozzarella, tofu cheese, etc.)

1/3 cup (180 mL) parmesan
   (dairy or soy)

1. Slice the zucchinis lengthwise (and cut off the stems). Scoop out the pulp, leaving a thin shell, but not so thin that it will break. If the seeds are large, dispose of them, but small, immature seeds are fine. The amount of pulp you end up with will vary depending on the zucchinis (we ended up with 2 cups [480 mL]). Place the zucchini shells in an oiled baking pan.

2. Chop the zucchini pulp fine and place it in a mixing bowl.

3. Sauté the leeks in olive oil. Remove from heat and add them and all the other ingredients (except the parmesan) to the bowl with the zucchini pulp. Mix well.

4. Fill the zucchini shells with the mixture and sprinkle the tops with the parmesan.

5. Cover the baking pan with foil and bake at 375°F (190°C) for 40 to 50 minutes. Then uncover the pan and continue baking for another 10 to 15 minutes until the zucchinis are soft and the parmesan begins to brown.

caribbean black beans

SERVES 8–10

Spicy but not hot. A surprising blend of ingredients makes this a taste treat with a charming Caribbean flavour. Serve with salsa.

1. Soak the beans overnight, then drain them.
2. Cover the beans with fresh water and bring them to a boil. Simmer 45 to 60 minutes or until the beans are soft, then strain, and discard the water.
3. Sauté the leeks and green peppers in 4 tablespoons (60 mL) olive oil.
4. Sauté the carrots (separately from the leeks and peppers) in 3 tablespoons (45 mL) olive oil, until they're cooked but still firm.
5. Sauté the spices in a separate pan in 4 tablespoons (60 mL) olive oil, then add the tomatoes. Cook until the tomatoes are soft.
6. In a large bowl, mix the beans, vegetables, and sautéd tomatoes and spices with the remaining ingredients.
7. Remove 2 cups (480 mL) of the mixture and purée it in a blender or food processor. Then return it to the bowl and mix it in.
8. Pour the mixture into a baking pan or casserole dish and cover it with foil.
9. Bake at 375°F (190°C) for 30 to 40 minutes.

3 1/2 cups (840 mL) dry black beans
Water to cover beans
11 Tbsp (165 mL) olive oil
3 cups (720 mL) chopped leeks
1 cup (240 mL) chopped green peppers
2 cups (480 mL) finely chopped carrots
2 Tbsp (30 mL) cumin
1 Tbsp (15 mL) coriander
1 Tbsp (15 mL) paprika
1 1/2 tsp (7 mL) salt
1/2 tsp (2 mL) pepper
1 cup (240 mL) chopped tomatoes
1 cup (240 mL) orange juice
3/4 cup (180 mL) finely minced fresh parsley
Pinch cayenne

curried garbanzo rice

A tasty, balanced full meal with a mild spicy flavour.

1 3/4 cups (420 mL) uncooked
   garbanzo beans
1 1/2 cups (360 mL) uncooked
   basmati rice
2 tsp (10 mL) cumin seeds
1 tsp (5 mL) coriander seeds
1/4 cup (60 mL) olive oil
3 cups (720 mL) chopped leeks
5 tsp (25 mL) curry powder
2 tsp (10 mL) cumin powder
1/2 tsp (2 mL) salt
1/2 tsp (2 mL) pepper
1/2 cup (120 mL) tamari

1. Cook the garbanzo beans in 5 1/4 cups (1.3 L) boiling water for 45 to 60 minutes or until the garbanzos are soft.

2. Cook the rice in 4 1/2 cups (1.08 L) of water for 15 to 20 minutes.

3. In a frying pan over medium-high heat, dry roast the cumin and coriander seeds until they pop. Add the olive oil and leeks, and sauté until the leeks cook down.

4. Add the other spices and tamari and mix in.

5. Add the garbanzo beans and cook for about 20 minutes, or until the garbanzos absorb the flavour of the spices.

6. Add the rice and mix it in, heating thoroughly.

win's banana curry

SERVES 4–6

A deliciously warming curry to enjoy on a cold winter day. You can adjust the amount of chili if you prefer a less spicy version.

1. Peel the bananas and cut them in half lengthwise. Sprinkle them with the salt and turmeric.

2. Fry the bananas in ghee for 2 minutes on each side.

3. In another pan, combine the coconut milk, nutmeg, chilies, fenugreek, fennel seeds, cinnamon stick, and curry leaves. Simmer over medium-low heat for approximately 30 to 40 minutes.

4. Add the bananas and cook, uncovered, over low heat for another 10 to 15 minutes.

5. Remove the cinnamon stick before serving.

4–6 large unripe bananas

1 tsp (5 mL) salt

1 tsp (5 mL) ground turmeric

5–6 Tbsp (75–90 mL) ghee (page 41)

2 cups (480 mL) coconut milk

1/4 tsp (1 mL) ground nutmeg

2 small, finely chopped fresh green or red chilies (stems and seeds removed)

1 tsp (5 mL) ground fenugreek (methi)

1/2 tsp (2 mL) crushed fennel seeds

2-inch (5 cm) piece cinnamon stick

4–5 curry leaves (if available)

A STROKE OF SERENDIPITY brought us this recipe. Nayana, on a visit to Salt Spring, raved about the cooking of her friend Win. Sharada called Win, who was only too happy to share her recipes. Although we still haven't met her except by phone, one day we'll get to meet and cook together.

eastern star curry

SERVES 6

To be enjoyed in a warm environment with friends, love, and laughter ... and a little rice!

1-inch ball (2.5 cm) tamarind pulp (or use mashed dates and dried apricots)

1/2 cup (120 mL) warm water

2-inch piece (5 cm) fresh ginger

1 Tbsp (15 mL) garam masala

1/2 tsp (2 mL) cardamom seeds

1 1/2 tsp (7 mL) coriander seeds

1 1/2 tsp (7 mL) cumin seeds

1/4 tsp (1 mL) ground nutmeg

4 whole black peppercorns

1 tsp (5 mL) ground turmeric

1 tsp (5 mL) fenugreek (methi)

2–3 finely minced fresh green or red chilies (stems and seeds removed)

4 Tbsp (60 mL) ghee (page 41)

1 Tbsp (15 mL) black mustard seeds

3–4 curry leaves (if available)

1. Dissolve the tamarind pulp in 1/2 cup (120 mL) of warm water for 10 minutes. Then strain. Discard the pulp and reserve the liquid.

2. Combine the ginger, garam masala, cardamom seeds, coriander seeds, cumin seeds, nutmeg, peppercorns, turmeric, fenugreek, and chilies in a food processor. Blend until the mixture forms a smooth paste. Add 1 to 2 teaspoons (5 to 10 mL) water if the mixture is too thick.

3. Heat the ghee over medium heat in a large heavy-bottomed pot (big enough for all the ingredients). Add the mustard seeds. When the seeds begin to pop, add the spice mixture that you blended and the curry leaves. Sauté for 3 to 5 minutes.

4. Add the chopped vegetables to the pot and mix them in with the spices, making sure the vegetables are well coated. Stir constantly for about 2 minutes.

5. Add the coconut milk and water, and mix well.

6. Cover and cook for half an hour.

7. Add the tamarind liquid and the tomatoes.

8. Reduce the heat to low and simmer, covered, for 45 minutes to 1 hour.

9. Add the mashed banana, raisins, and apricots. Continue to simmer on low heat for another 30 to 45 minutes.

10. Add the almonds. Add salt to taste. Garnish with the fresh mint leaves.

6 cups (1.54 L) chopped vegetables
(yams, cauliflower, broccoli, green
beans, carrots, peppers, squash,
or eggplant)

3 cups (720 mL) coconut milk

1 1/2 cups (360 mL) water

2 chopped ripe tomatoes

1 mashed ripe banana

1/2 cup (120 mL) raisins

1/2 cup (120 mL) chopped
dried apricots

1/3 cup (80 mL) almonds

1/3 cup (80 mL) coarsely chopped
fresh mint leaves

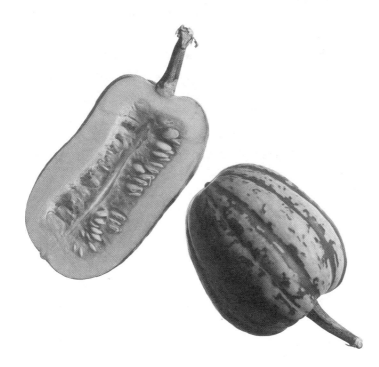

ramanand's dal

This is definitely not dull dal! Serve as an accompaniment to your favourite curry.

2 cups (480 mL) red lentils

6 1/2 cups (1.56 L) water

1 tsp (5 mL) salt

1/3 cup (80 mL) ghee (page 41)

1 Tbsp (15 mL) black mustard seeds

1 cup (240 mL) finely chopped leeks

1 heaping Tbsp (15–20 mL) grated
 fresh ginger

2 heaping Tbsp (30–35 mL) ground
 coriander

2 heaping Tbsp (30–35 mL) ground
 cumin

1/2 tsp (2 mL) ground fenugreek

1 heaping Tbsp (15–20 mL) curry
 powder

1/2 tsp (2 mL) ground cardamom

1 heaping tsp (5–8 mL) chili powder

1 heaping Tbsp (15–20 mL) garam
 masala

1. Wash and strain the lentils, removing any pebbles or twigs. Cook the lentils in the water. Bring to a rapid boil, then turn the heat down and simmer until the lentils are soft. Add the salt.

2. In a frying pan, cook the mustard seeds in the ghee on fairly high heat until they pop, then add the leeks and ginger.

3. Turn the heat down and add all the spices except the garam masala. Sauté until the leeks are cooked, then add the garam masala and mix it in.

4. Stir the spice mixture into the cooked lentils.

ghee

A.k.a. clarified butter. Once the milk solids are removed, ghee keeps beautifully at room temperature for many months.

1. Heat the butter over low heat so that it doesn't brown. When it's all melted, let it sit, preferably in a cool spot, then skim off all the whitish milk solids that accumulate on top. Pour it through a fine strainer or a few layers of cheesecloth to remove the last bits of solids.

2. Pour the golden ghee into a wide-mouth jar.

1 lb (454 g) butter

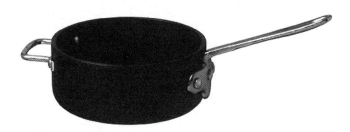

kitcheree

SERVES 8–10

Kitcheree is a combination of mung beans, rice, and spices that warms and nourishes, and just plain tastes good. You can make it thick or soupy, to your taste.

6 Tbsp (90 mL) ghee (page 41)

1/2 tsp (2 mL) black mustard seeds

1 Tbsp (15 mL) turmeric

2 tsp (10 mL) coriander

3 Tbsp (45 mL) cumin

1/2–1 tsp (2–5 mL) chili flakes

1–2 tsp (5–10 mL) salt

1 cup (240 mL) chopped leeks

1 cup (240 mL) split mung beans
   (uncooked)

1 cup (480 mL) basmati rice
   (uncooked)

8 cups (1.92 L) water

5 Tbsp (75 mL) ginger juice
   (see tips)

1. Heat the ghee in a soup pot. When it's hot, add the mustard seeds. When they pop, add the other spices (except ginger) and the leeks.

2. Stir the spices for a minute or two. Watch that they don't burn.

3. Add the rice and mung beans. Stir to coat them with the spices. Then add the water and bring it to a boil. Cover the pot and turn the heat down to simmer until the rice and mung beans are cooked (about half an hour).

4. Add the ginger juice.

5. You can add more water if you prefer your kitcheree soupier, and more ghee if you want it richer.

TIPS   PERFECT FOOD/GINGER JUICE

• Kitcheree is an example of a perfect food; Ayurveda says that it is balanced for all doshas. For those times when you feel out of balance, kitcheree is the perfect food for you. The problem is that when you're feeling ungrounded, your mind races and you can't relax, so you may not be inclined to cook something that's good for you (or even think of it). Perhaps a sticky note on the fridge might help: Do you need kitcheree today?

• To make ginger juice, grate a piece of fresh ginger (the fresher the better) and squeeze the grated ginger over a cup or bowl.

leah's chai

MAKES 9 CUPS (2.16 L)

In India *chai* means tea, and there are as many variations as there are tea sellers. This is Leah's special version. Dry roasting the tea before adding it improves the flavour and reduces the tannic acid, though it isn't necessary.

1. Pour the water into a pot and add the cinnamon, cardamom, peppercorns, and ginger.
2. Bring it to a boil and let it simmer for half an hour.
3. In a separate pot, scald the milk, and set it aside.
4. Dry roast the tea in a frying pan over low heat just until it begins to move.
5. Add the tea and sugar to the spice water. Bring it to the boiling point, but don't boil it.
6. Remove the tea bags (if using), strain the tea, and pour the strained tea back into the pot.
7. Add the scalded milk and bring to a rolling boil, very briefly.

6 cups (1.54 L) water

1 cinnamon stick

1 heaping Tbsp (15–20 mL) cardamom seeds or 2 heaping Tbsp (30–35 mL) cardamom seeds in the pod

1/4 tsp (1 mL) whole black peppercorns

1/4–1/2 cup (60–120 mL) finely sliced ginger

3 cups (720 mL) milk

6–8 tsp (30–40 mL) loose black tea or 4 black tea bags

1/3 cup (80 mL) turbinado sugar

TIPS VARIATIONS

- Variations: Try adding anise seeds or cloves.
- You can make chai with soy or rice milk, too—but in that case, heat the milk and don't scald it.
- If you like your chai foamy, blend it before serving.

sweet and sour tofu

SERVES 8–10

A taste of China in your own home.

2 lb (1 kg) tofu
2 Tbsp (30 mL) olive oil
1/3 cup (80 mL) tamari or Bragg's
    (page 10)

Sauce:
1 1/2–2 Tbsp (17–30 mL) grated
    ginger
1/2 cup and 2 Tbsp (150 mL)
    turbinado sugar
1 cup (240 mL) cider vinegar
2 Tbsp (30 mL) tamari
6 oz (170 g) tomato paste
2 Tbsp (30 mL) arrowroot powder
    mixed in 1/4 cup (60 mL) water

1. Cut the tofu into 1/4-inch (0.5 cm) slices. Cut each slice diagonally to make triangles.
2. Brown the tofu in a frying pan with the olive oil and tamari or Bragg's.
3. Place all the sauce ingredients in a saucepan and bring to a boil, then simmer until the sugar dissolves and the sauce begins to thicken.
4. Place the tofu in a baking pan and cover it with the sauce.
5. Bake at 350°F (180°C) for 45 minutes.

mexican lasagna

A quicker version of enchiladas. Serve with yogurt or sour cream.

1. In a large bowl, combine the beans, tomatoes, corn, leeks, chilies, and spices.
2. Grate the cheese in a separate bowl.
3. Oil a baking pan (8 x 8 inch [20 x 20 cm] or 9 x 12 inch [23 x 30 cm]) and line it with 4 corn tortillas (or 6 if your pan is larger), overlapping them if necessary.
4. Spread half the bean-corn mixture over the tortillas.
5. Sprinkle the mixture with half the cheese.
6. Repeat with the remaining tortillas, bean-corn mixture, and cheese.
7. Bake at 375°F (190°C) for half an hour.

2 cups (480 mL) cooked and drained beans (kidney, pinto, or black beans)

2 cups (480 mL) crushed canned tomatoes

2 cups (480 mL) frozen corn

1 cup (240 mL) chopped leeks

4-oz tin (112 g) chopped green chilies

1/2 tsp (2 mL) salt

1 Tbsp (15 mL) oregano

1 Tbsp (15 mL) cumin

1/2 tsp (2 mL) chili flakes (optional—or use more if you want it spicier)

2 cups (480 mL) grated cheese (cheddar or soy)

8–12 corn tortillas (depending on size of pan)

SOME OF OUR RECIPES COME TO US IN UNEXPECTED WAYS. Leandre was back at the Centre for a second visit. During dinner on Saturday, she was chatting with some of us about food (a subject that comes up frequently during meals) and mentioned that she had a great recipe she'd love to contribute to our new book, saying that for a period of time her daughter would eat nothing else. A short while later, a fax arrived with this recipe. Thanks again Leandre!

spicy tofu tostadas

SERVES 8–10

If you can't get to Mexico, bring Mexico to you!

2 Tbsp (30 mL) olive oil

4 cups (960 mL) cubed tofu

2 Tbsp (30 mL) tamari or Bragg's
(page 10)

1/2 tsp (2 mL) salt

2–4 Tbsp (15–60 mL) juice from
pickled jalapeno peppers

2 cups (480 mL) chopped green
peppers

2 cups (480 mL) chopped zucchini

1/4 cup (60 mL) pitted and sliced
Greek olives

2 cups (480 mL) sliced mushrooms

1 cup (240 mL) chopped tomatoes

1–1 1/2 cups (240–360 mL) finely
chopped pickled jalapeno peppers

1 Tbsp (15 mL) balsamic vinegar

1. On medium-high heat, brown the tofu in olive oil with the Bragg's or tamari, salt, and juice from the jar of pickled jalapenos. Keep stirring the tofu until it browns on all sides.

2. When the tofu is browned, add the green peppers, zucchini, and olives. Stir until the vegetables begin to soften.

3. Add the mushrooms, tomatoes, jalapeno peppers, and balsamic vinegar. Keep stirring until the liquid is gone.

4. Serve this spicy mixture on toasted corn tortillas or on a bed of rice, with chopped lettuce and a dab of yogurt or sour cream.

risotto

A far more interesting way to deal with rice and veggies—and very pretty too!
(Not to mention delicious.)

Stock:
1. Put all the ingredients for the stock into a pot and bring to a boil. Partially cover and simmer for 40 to 45 minutes. Then strain it, reserve the liquid, and discard the rest.

Vegetable and Rice:
1. Sauté the leeks in olive oil until they're soft, then add the uncooked rice. Stir for 5 minutes over medium-low heat until the rice becomes translucent.
2. Add 1 cup (240 mL) of stock and stir until the stock is absorbed into the rice. Keep adding the stock and stirring, 1 cup (240 mL) at a time, until you've used all the stock.
3. Add the veggies, cover, and turn the heat down to low. Simmer 5 to 10 minutes more until the rice is cooked but not mushy, and the vegetables are cooked.
4. Add the pepper and parmesan at the end.

Stock:
8 cups (1.92 L) water
3 cups (720 mL) chopped leeks
3 cups (720 mL) chopped carrots
2 cups (720 mL) chopped celery
2 bay leaves
1/2 tsp (2 mL) salt
2 tsp (10 mL) pepper

Vegetable and Rice:
2 cups (480 mL) chopped leeks
1/4 cup (60 mL) olive oil
2 cups (480 mL) uncooked basmati rice
1 1/2 cups (360 mL) sliced green beans
3 cups (720 mL) chopped zucchini
1 cup (240 mL) chopped green peppers
1/2 tsp (2 mL) pepper
1/2– 3/4 cup (120–180 mL) parmesan cheese

spanakopita

This isn't as difficult as you may think. It just takes a little extra time—and it's worth every mouthful! You won't use a whole box of filo pastry, but it can be refrozen if it's carefully rolled back up.

6 cups (1.54 L) chopped spinach
  (2 bunches)

1 cup (240 mL) chopped leeks

1–1 1/2 cups (240–360 mL) crumbled
  or grated feta

1/4–1/2 tsp (1–2 mL) salt

1/4 tsp (1 mL) pepper

2 tsp (10 mL) dillweed

7 sheets filo pastry

1/3–1/2 cup (80–120 mL) melted
butter, olive oil or ghee (page 41)

1. Steam the spinach and leeks until the spinach is soft. Remove it from the heat and place it in a bowl.

2. Add the feta and spices, and mix everything together.

3. Cut the filo pastry into rectangles of approximately 5 1/2 x 13 1/2 inches (14 x 34 cm) (the width of the filo). You can get about 3 rectangles from one sheet of filo. If you end up with strips of the wrong size, you can patch them together. It won't show.

4. Place one of these filo rectangles on a counter or cutting board and brush it with ghee or olive oil. Then lay a second rectangle over the first and brush it with ghee or oil. Repeat this 2 more times so you have 4 layers of filo pastry rectangles, each brushed with ghee or oil.

5. Place a spoonful of the spinach mixture in one corner.

6. Fold the edges over the filling.

7. Fold the bottom left corner of the filo diagonally over the filling, making a small triangle.

8. Keep folding over and over, keeping the triangle shape, until you've reached the end. Tuck the ends under (like making a bed).

9. Place the spanakopitas on a baking tray and brush them with more ghee or oil.

10. Bake at 350°F (180°C) until they're golden brown—about 20 to 25 minutes.

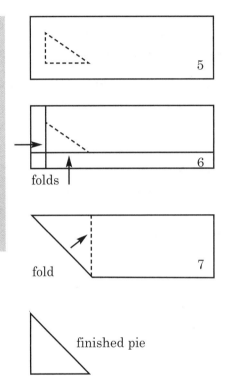

folds

fold

finished pie

TIPS PATCHING FILO

• While you're getting the knack of it, you may find you have pieces that need patching. Don't worry—patching is okay. As long as the patching isn't on the outer layer, it won't show anyway.

scott's samosas

SERVES 12 OR MORE AS A SIDE DISH

These samosas are a great part of an Indian dinner. For a dairy-free version, replace the yogurt in the dough with olive oil. Other vegetables can be used in place of yams, carrots, and peas. Try corn and potatoes for a change.

Dough:

1/4 cup (60 mL) olive oil or
   ghee (page 41)
1/4 cup (60 mL) plain yogurt
1/2 Tbsp (7.5 mL) salt
3 cups (720 mL) whole wheat
   pastry flour
1/2–3/4 cup (120–180 mL) water

1. In a bowl or measuring cup, mix the oil, yogurt, and salt until blended.
2. Place the flour in a mixing bowl and add the oil-yogurt-salt mixture. Mix with a fork until the dough is crumbly.
3. Gradually add warm water (up to 3/4 cup [180 mL]) until the dough forms a ball but is still slightly sticky. Do not overmix.
4. Sauté the leeks in olive oil.
5. Add the salt, pepper, and spices to the leeks, stirring until the leeks are soft. Set this mixture aside.
6. Place the yams and carrots in a pot with 1/2 cup water. Bring to a boil, cover, turn heat down to low, and simmer for about 15 minutes, or until the vegetables are soft.
7. Turn off the heat and add the peas, leek and spice mixture, ginger juice, and cilantro. Stir well.

TIPS   SAMOSAS

• If you make a big batch, you can keep some in the fridge for a scrumptious quick lunch. They also freeze well.

Assembly:

1. Flour a board or counter, and roll out the dough until it is fairly thin.

2. Using a bowl of 6 or 7 inches (15 to 18 cm) in diameter, cut circles in the dough. Then cut each circle in half.

3. Holding a semi-circular piece of dough in one hand, dip one finger of your other hand into a bowl of water, and moisten the edges of the dough. This will help the edges stick together.

4. Add about 2 tablespoons of filling to one side of the dough wrapper.

5. Folding the other side of the dough wrapper over the top of the filling, pinch the edges together, making sure the filling doesn't leak out. (If it does, the samosa will tend to split while it's baking.) Repeat.

6. Place the samosas on an oiled cookie sheet, and brush the tops with oil or ghee.

7. Bake at 350°F (180°C) 30 to 45 minutes, or until the samosas begin to brown.

Filling:

3 cups (720 mL) minced leeks

2 Tbsp (30 mL) olive oil

1/2 tsp (2 mL) salt

1/4 tsp (1 mL) pepper

1 tsp (5 mL) ground coriander

1 tsp (5 mL) ground cumin

2 tsp (10 mL) curry powder

1/4 tsp (1 mL) cayenne

3 cups (720 mL) peeled and diced yams

2 cups (480 mL) diced carrots

1/2 cup (120 mL) water

1 1/2 cup (360 mL) frozen peas

2 Tbsp (30 mL) fresh ginger juice (see sidebar)

1/4 cup (60 mL) minced fresh cilantro

TIPS   GINGER JUICE

• To make ginger juice, grate fresh ginger (about 1/2 cup [120 ml]) and squeeze the grated ginger over a cup or bowl.

the beet goes on!

SERVES 12 OR MORE AS A SIDE DISH

Served chilled as an accompaniment. These sweet and sour beets are very attractive and work well with many different meals, especially those that look good in magenta.

6 cups (1.54 L) peeled and sliced
   beets

Sauce:
1/2 cup (120 mL) balsamic vinegar
1/4 cup (60 mL) turbinado sugar
2 Tbsp (30 mL) maple syrup
2 Tbsp (30 mL) arrowroot powder
1 cup (240 mL) water

1. Steam the beets for 15 to 20 minutes or until tender, and set aside.
2. In a saucepan, bring the vinegar, sugar, and maple syrup to a boil, then reduce the heat and simmer until the sugar dissolves.
3. Mix the arrowroot with the water and add it to the vinegar, sugar, and syrup mixture. Stir until it thickens.
4. Pour the sauce over the beets and refrigerate to let them marinate. The longer they marinate, the more the beets absorb the flavour. You could serve them after an hour or leave them overnight.
5. Serve with a bit of the marinade poured over.

creole aubergine

SERVES 4–6 AS A SIDE DISH

This recipe accompanied the first settlers to Louisiana from France centuries ago. Naturally, they travelled with their eggplants.

1. Peel and dice the eggplant, set it in a colander, and sprinkle it generously with salt. Set it aside for 15 minutes.
2. In a frying pan, sauté the leeks and peppers in olive oil until they soften. Stir in the flour.
3. Add the tomatoes and tamari. Cook over medium heat for 10 to 15 minutes or until the tomatoes are soft.
4. Add the 1/2–1 teaspoon salt, plus the pepper, sugar, and parsley.
5. Take the frying pan ingredients off the heat while you rinse the eggplant and steam it until it is soft.
6. Drain the eggplant and put it in a mixing bowl with the sautéed mixture and toss well. Oil a casserole dish and pour the eggplant mixture into it. Sprinkle with parmesan cheese.
7. Bake, uncovered, at 350°F (180°C) for 30 minutes.

1 medium eggplant
Salt
3 Tbsp (45 mL) olive oil
1 1/2 cups (360 mL) chopped leeks
1 cup (240 mL) diced green, red, or yellow peppers
4 Tbsp (60 mL) flour
4 cups (960 mL) diced fresh tomatoes
1 Tbsp (15 mL) tamari
1/2–1 tsp (2–5 mL) salt
1/2 tsp (2 mL) pepper
2 Tbsp (30 mL) turbinado sugar
1/2 cup (120 mL) finely minced parsley
1/4 cup (60 mL) parmesan

WE HAVE TO ADMIT THAT THE INTRODUCTION to this recipe is only there to get your attention. In fact, this recipe was inspired by Sharada's mom, who, at the age of 82, is still a fabulous cook. In addition to cooking, she paints and gardens. Here's to you, Julie!

ginger-tamari roasted mushrooms

SERVES 4 AS AN APPETIZER OR SIDE DISH

Mushrooms become a delicacy when cooked this way. Try them! You'll never go back to ordinary mushrooms again.

12 cups (2.9 L) whole mushrooms

Sauce:
3/4 cup (180 mL) tamari
2 Tbsp (30 mL) grated ginger
1/4 cup (60 mL) finely minced leeks
2 Tbsp (30 mL) olive oil

1. Wash the mushrooms and set aside in a bowl.
2. Assemble the sauce by whisking together the ingredients.
3. Pour the sauce over the mushrooms to marinate them (uncooked) for 15 to 20 minutes. Mix well to make sure they're well coated.
4. In a large skillet, roast the mushrooms with the sauce over medium-high heat, starting with the tops of the mushrooms down.
5. As you allow the liquid to boil off, keep rotating the mushrooms. When the button tops are browned, turn them on their sides so they brown all over. They should be softened but not overheated. This takes about 15 minutes.
6. Serve immediately. Delicious served over rice.

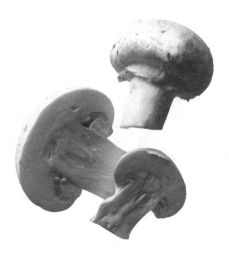

green bean curry

SERVES 4 AS A SIDE DISH

One of the best uses for green beans in season, especially if your garden over-produced and your friends won't take any more. A nice marriage of sweetness and spice.

1. In a saucepan or deep frying pan sauté the leeks in 4 tablespoons (60 mL) ghee or oil. Add the beans and sauté for a few minutes, then add the water, cover, and let the beans steam.

2. Meanwhile, heat the remaining ghee or oil in another pan over medium-low heat and add the spices, including the ginger and salt, but not the garam masala.

3. Stir the spices carefully for a minute or so. Keep stirring to make sure the mixture doesn't burn.

4. Add the coconut milk to the spice mixture and let it cook for a few minutes. Add the garam masala and mix it in.

5. Pour the spice and coconut milk mixture over the beans and stir.

6. Cook over low heat until the beans are soft and the flavours are blended.

2 cups (480 mL) chopped leeks
6 cups (1.54 L) sliced green beans
6 Tbsp (90 mL) ghee (page 41) or oil
1/2 cup (120 mL) water
1 Tbsp (15 mL) cumin
2 tsp (10 mL) coriander
2 tsp (10 mL) chili powder
2 tsp (10 mL) turmeric
3 Tbsp (45 mL) grated ginger
1 tsp (5 mL) salt
13.5-oz tin (400 mL) coconut milk
1 Tbsp (15 mL) garam masala

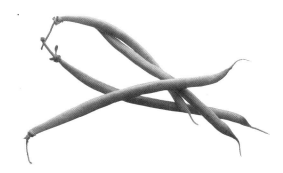

zesty ginger beans

SERVES 4 AS A SIDE DISH

Use any kind of snap beans you like, but they must be fresh. Even if your garden has run amuck with beans and you never want to see another, this recipe will have you back in the bean patch in no time.

5 cups (1.2 L) fresh green or yellow
  beans
1/4 cup (60 mL) thinly sliced ginger
4 Tbsp (60 mL) vegetable oil or
  olive oil
5 Tbsp (75 mL) tamari
1/4 cup (60 mL) water
1 Tbsp (15 mL) fresh lemon juice

1. Slice the beans into approximately 2-inch (5-cm) lengths, removing both ends of the beans.

2. In a frying pan, sauté the beans and ginger in oil for 3 to 4 minutes.

4. Add the tamari, water, and lemon juice.

5. Reduce the heat, cover, and simmer until the beans are cooked.

mary's ginger yams

SERVES 4–6 AS A SIDE DISH

A very popular item at Centre meals and one of many recipes created by Mary, an excellent cook who graced our kitchen for many months

1. Dry roast the cumin seeds over medium-low heat until they pop.
2. Sauté the leeks and ginger in ghee, butter, or oil.
3. Add the yams and continue to sauté on medium-low heat for 15 minutes, or until the yams begin to soften.
4. Add the Bragg's or tamari and the cumin seeds and mix them in.
5. Place the yams in a baking pan and bake uncovered at 400°F (205°C) for 20 to 25 minutes, or until the yams are soft and slightly browned.

3 Tbsp (45 mL) cumin seeds

2 cups (480 mL) finely minced leeks

5 Tbsp (75 mL) finely minced ginger

6 cups (1.54 L) peeled and cubed yams

4 Tbsp (60 mL) ghee (page 41), butter, or vegetable oil

5 Tbsp (75 mL) Bragg's (page 10) or 3 Tbsp (45 mL) tamari

sweet cinnamon yams

SERVES 4–6 AS A SIDE DISH

So easy, so sweet … mmm!

6 cups (1.54 L) thinly sliced yams
6 Tbsp (90 mL) vegetable oil
1 1/2 Tbsp (22 mL) cinnamon
Pinch cayenne

1. Toss all the ingredients in a mixing bowl until the yams are well covered.
2. Place the yams in a greased casserole dish and bake, uncovered, at 400°F (205°C) for half an hour, or until the yams are soft.

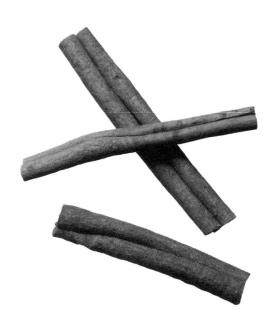

roasted reds

You probably think this dish is much too time-consuming to make at home, but surprise! This recipe shows you how easy red peppers are to prepare, and how delicious they are too. Serve with pita or focaccia bread.

1. Roast the red peppers whole under the broiler until the skins start to turn black. Keep rotating them, watching that they don't burn. Then take them out of the oven and allow them to cool only enough so that you can handle them.
2. Peel the skins off and remove the seeds. Slice the peppers into thin strips.
3. Mix the dressing ingredients together and pour the mixture over the peppers.
4. Refrigerate. It's best if they sit overnight.

3 large red peppers

Dressing:
1/4 cup (60 mL) balsamic vinegar
2 Tbsp (30 mL) olive oil
1/2 cup (120 mL) crumbled feta
1 Tbsp (15 mL) oregano
1/2 tsp (2 mL) salt
1/2 tsp (2 mL) pepper

roasted roots

An easy, warming meal that prepares itself while you finish writing the Great Canadian Novel. Use any combination you like of your favourite root vegetables.

2 cups (480 mL) coarsely chopped leeks

2–2 1/2 cups (480–600 mL) chopped potatoes

2–2 1/2 cups (480–600 mL) chopped yams

2 cups (480 mL) chopped carrots

1 Tbsp (15 mL) oregano

1 Tbsp (15 mL) basil

1 Tbsp (15 mL) parsley

1 tsp (5 mL) rosemary

1/2–1 tsp (2–5 mL) salt

1/2 tsp (2 mL) pepper

1. In a bowl, sprinkle the spices over the vegetables and mix in.

2. Spread out the chopped vegetables in an oiled baking pan or on a cookie sheet.

3. Cover the pan and bake at 400°F (205°C) for 45 minutes.

4. Uncover the pan and bake 15 minutes more or until the vegetables are soft and beginning to brown.

scalloped potatoes

An oldie, but goodie; this non-dairy version will thrill those with dairy allergies (although you can make a dairy version, too).

1. Slice the potatoes thin and lay half the potatoes, overlapping, on the bottom of an oiled casserole dish.
2. Sprinkle half the leeks over the potatoes, then half of each of the following: parsley, flour, cheddar or tofu cheese, parmesan cheese, salt, and pepper.
3. Make another layer of potatoes over the first layer.
4. Add the milk or soymilk, then top this with the remaining leeks, parsley, flour, salt, pepper, and cheese.
5. Sprinkle the top with the 3 tablespoons parmesan.
6. Cover the casserole dish and bake at 375°F (190°C) for 1 hour. Then uncover it and let it bake for a few more minutes until the top begins to brown.

6 medium potatoes
2–3 Tbsp (30–45 mL) olive oil
1 cup (240 mL) finely minced leeks
1/2 cup (120 mL) finely minced parsley
2 Tbsp (30 mL) flour
2 cups (480 mL) cheddar or tofu cheese
2 cups (480 mL) parmesan (dairy or soy)
1/2–1 tsp (2–5 mL) salt
1/2–1tsp (2–5 mL) pepper or pinch cayenne
2 cups (480 mL) milk or soymilk
3 Tbsp (45 mL) parmesan

well-dressed potatoes

SERVES 6

Stuffed with a delicious filling into their jackets, making them the best-dressed potatoes in town. Serve with a salad for a simple lunch or as part of *un grand dîner.*

3 large baking potatoes

1/4–1/3 cup (60–80 mL) butter
  or ghee (page 00)

1/2 cup (120 mL) chopped leeks

1 cup (240 mL) yogurt or sour cream

1/2–1 tsp (2–5 mL) salt

1/2 tsp (2 mL) pepper

1 cup (240 mL) grated cheddar or
  tofu cheese

Paprika as a garnish

1. Prick the potatoes with a fork. Rub them with oil if desired.
2. Bake them at 400°F (205°C) for about 75 to 80 minutes. Then allow them to cool to the touch.
3. Cut the potatoes in half lengthwise.
4. Carefully scoop out the pulp, leaving a thin shell. Place the pulp in a mixing bowl and mash it well.
5. Sauté the leeks in butter or ghee until tender. Add them to the pulp, along with the yogurt or sour cream, salt, and pepper.
6. Fold in the grated cheese.
7. Stuff the mixture into the potato shells and place them in a 9 x 13 inch (23 x 33 cm) baking pan. Sprinkle the tops with paprika.
8. Bake at 350°F (180°C) for 20 to 30 minutes.

TIPS TIMESAVER

• This recipe can be prepared and cooked ahead of time and refrigerated or frozen (make sure you allow additional time for reheating).

zucchini feta

A nice, easy Mediterranean vegetable dish—wonderful served over rice.

1. In a frying pan, sauté the leeks in olive oil until soft. Add the zucchini, tomatoes, tamari, and spices, and mix in.

2. Cover the pan and cook over low heat until the zucchinis are soft. Remove the pan from the heat, and mix in the feta just before serving.

2 cups (480 mL) chopped leeks

4 Tbsp (60 mL) olive oil

7 cups (1.68 L) diced zucchini

2 1/2 cups (600 mL) chopped tomatoes

2 Tbsp (30 mL) tamari

1 1/2 Tbsp (22 mL) oregano

1 Tbsp (15 mL) basil

1/2 tsp (5 mL) pepper

1 1/2–2 cups (360–480 mL) crumbled feta

daya's quinoa salad

SERVES 4–6

If you've never tried quinoa (a protein-rich native of South America) or you think you don't like it, try this delightful and unusual combination of textures and temperatures.

1/2–3/4 cup (120–180 mL) sundried tomatoes

1 1/2 cups (360 mL) water

1 cup (240 mL) quinoa

8 Tbsp (120 mL) olive oil

1 1/2 cups (360 mL) chopped leeks

3 cups (720 mL) sliced mushrooms

2 cups (480 mL) diced zucchini

1 cup (240 mL) sliced artichoke hearts

1/4 cup (60 mL) oil from the artichoke hearts

1/3–1/2 cup (80–120 mL) balsamic vinegar

5 Tbsp (75 mL) Bragg's (page 10)

1/2 tsp (2 mL) salt

1/2 tsp (2 mL) pepper

4 cups (960 mL) baby salad greens (optional)

1/3–1/2 cup (80–120 mL) finely minced chives (optional)

1. Soak the sundried tomatoes in boiling water while you prepare the other ingredients.
2. Rinse the quinoa in a strainer under running water for at least 5 minutes. (If it's not well rinsed, it will be bitter.)
3. When it's well rinsed, pat the quinoa dry with a dish towel. Then dry roast it over low heat until it becomes aromatic and begins to pop and turn just a bit brown.
4. Place toasted quinoa in a saucepan with 1 1/2 cups water. Bring to a boil, then reduce heat, cover and simmer for 15 to 20 minutes. Remove from heat and place in a large bowl.
5. Stir-fry the leeks, mushrooms, and zucchini in 4 tablespoons (60 mL) olive oil, then add them to the quinoa.
6. When the sundried tomatoes are soft, chop them into small pieces and add them to the quinoa.
7. Add the rest of the ingredients except the salad greens and chives, and toss well.
8. Serve as is, or if you prefer, mix in the greens and chives just before serving.

daya's summer salad

SERVES 6

Imagine a big bowl of fresh spinach sprinkled with asiago cheese, nuts, and dressing, glistening in the late afternoon sun. Very refreshing on a hot day. Try garnishing with fresh red raspberries.

1. Mix the dressing in a jar and set aside.
2. Wash the spinach, tear it into bite-size pieces, and pour the dressing over it.
3. Chop the pine nuts and sauté them in butter or ghee. Sprinkle them over the spinach greens.
4. Sprinkle the cheese on the salad, then toss.
5. Garnish with fresh raspberries in season.

Dressing:
1/4 cup (60 mL) olive oil
1/8 cup (30 mL) balsamic vinegar
1/8—1/4 cup (30–60 mL) maple syrup
1/4 tsp (1 mL) salt
1/4 tsp (1 mL) pepper

Salad:
8 cups (1.92 L) spinach
1/2 cup (120 mL) pine nuts or walnuts
1–2 Tbsp (15–30 mL) butter or ghee (page 41)
3/4 cup (180 mL) grated asiago cheese or fresh grated parmesan
Fresh raspberries (optional)

DAYA GREW UP AS PART OF the yoga community that became The Salt Spring Centre. She is an artist both in and out of the kitchen.

lebanese tabouli

SERVES 4–6

As close to authentic as we could make it. A Lebanese woman who visited the Centre said it tasted like home.

3/4 cup (180 mL) bulgur

3 1/2 cups (840 mL) boiling water

2 medium tomatoes, chopped into small pieces

1/3 cup (80 mL) finely minced leeks

2 cups (480 mL) finely minced parsley

4–5 Tbsp (60–75 mL) fresh lemon juice

1/2–1 tsp (2–5 mL) salt

3/4 cup (180 mL) olive oil

4 Tbsp (60 mL) finely minced fresh mint leaves

1. Soak the bulgur in the boiling water for 45 minutes, then strain and rinse with cold water.

2. Mix all the other ingredients together with the bulgur.

marinated mushroom salad

SERVES 6–8

An immediate hit! Goes well with any entrée of substance and good bearing, like a nut loaf or quiche.

1. Mix all the salad ingredients, except for the spinach.
2. Mix the dressing ingredients and pour it over the salad.
3. Refrigerate the salad for an hour or more so that it can marinate before serving.
4. Before serving, add the spinach and mix it in.

Salad:

4 cups (960 mL) thinly sliced mushrooms

1 cup (240 mL) thinly sliced celery

1 cup (240 mL) thinly sliced red or green peppers

1/4 cup (60 mL) finely minced leeks or chives

1/2 cup (120 mL) finely minced parsley

1/2 cup (120 mL) pitted and sliced Greek olives

1 cup (240 mL) sliced artichoke hearts

3 cups (720 mL) spinach

Dressing:

1/2 cup (120 mL) olive oil

1/3 cup (80 mL) balsamic or red wine vinegar

3 Tbsp (45 mL) lemon juice

2 tsp (10 mL) oregano

1/2 tsp (2 mL) salt

1/2 tsp (2 mL) pepper

1 Tbsp (15 mL) tamari

julie's nutty apricot pasta salad

SERVES 6-8

Fresh herbs make this pasta salad lively, and the apricots add a nice surprising sweetness. This recipe calls for rotini, but you can use your favourite pasta.

Salad:

5 cups (1.2 L) cooked rotini pasta

2 cups (480 mL) peppers (red, green, or yellow), cut into strips

1 cup (240 mL) grated carrots

1/3 cup (80 mL) finely minced leeks

1 1/2–2 cups (360–480 mL) crumbled feta

1/2 cup (120 mL) chopped apricots (dried or fresh)

1 cup (240 mL) pine nuts or sunflower seeds

Dressing:

1/2 cup (120 mL) olive oil

1/3 cup (80 mL) balsamic vinegar

1/2–1 Tbsp (7–15 mL) finely grated ginger

1/2 tsp (2 mL) salt (optional— depends on the saltiness of the feta)

1/2 cup (120 mL) finely minced fresh basil (or 1 Tbsp [15 mL] dried)

3/4 cup (180 mL) finely minced fresh dillweed (or 3 Tbsp [45 mL] dried)

1. Mix all the salad ingredients together.
2. Mix all the dressing ingredients together, pour over the salad, and mix it in.
3. Refrigerate, allowing the salad to marinate for a while before serving.

JULIE'S BEEN AN ACTIVELY INVOLVED PARENT AT the Salt Spring Centre School for several years. At the end of each school year, some of the parents prepare and serve a wonderful lunch for the staff. Julie's contribution last year was so good that we asked her if she'd contribute the recipe for the book.

mary's potato salad

Piquant and lively with a nice crunch. Sprinkle the top with paprika or dress with edible flowers. Let the flavours meld for at least half an hour before serving.

1. Peel (optional) and cube the potatoes. Steam them for about 20 minutes until they're soft but still firm. Then set them aside to cool.

2. When the potatoes have cooled, add all the other ingredients and mix everything together.

16 medium potatoes

2 cups (480 mL) finely minced leeks

1 1/3 cups (320 mL) finely minced celery

1 1/2 cups (360 mL) eggless mayonnaise

1 1/2 tsp (7 mL) dry mustard

3/4 tsp (3 mL) salt

1 tsp (5 mL) pepper

4 Tbsp (60 mL) dillweed

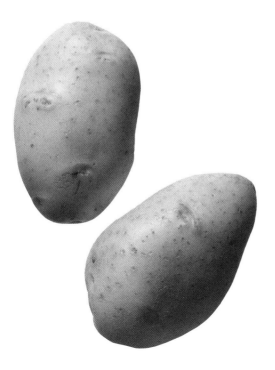

sunny day carrot salad

SERVES 6–8 AS A SIDE DISH

If it's not sunny outside, this salad will bring the sun to you!

5 cups (1.2 L) grated carrot

3 Tbsp (45 mL) finely minced leeks

1/2 cup (120 mL) finely minced parsley

1/4 cup (60 mL) sesame seeds

2–3 tsp (10–15 mL) finely grated ginger

2 Tbsp (30 mL) tamari

4 Tbsp (50 mL) fresh lemon juice

1/2 cup (120 mL) olive or vegetable oil (or half and half)

1/2 tsp (2 mL) salt

1/4–1/2 tsp (1–2 mL) pepper

1. Mix all the ingredients together and serve.

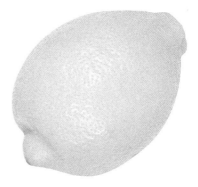

alicia's raspberry vinaigrette

MAKES 1 1/2 CUPS (360 ML)

Alicia, our youngest cook, brings us another unique recipe. Very pink, very tasty, very unusual over greens.

1. In a blender, combine all the ingredients until smooth.

1 cup (240 mL) fresh or frozen
  raspberries
1/2 cup (120 mL) olive oil
1/4 cup (60 mL) vinegar (apple cider
  or balsamic, or a combination)
1/2 cup (120 mL) orange juice
2 Tbsp (30 mL) chopped leeks
1/2– 3/4 tsp (2–3 mL) Dijon mustard
Small pinch rosemary
1/2 tsp (2 mL) basil
1/2 tsp (2 mL) dillweed

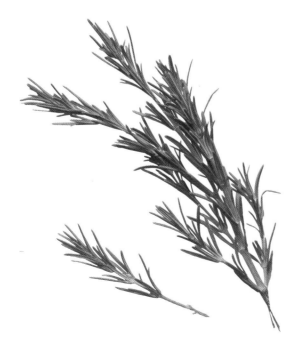

donna's maple balsamic dressing

MAKES 1 3/4 CUPS (420 ML)

Speaks for itself: quick, easy, and delicious.

1 cup (240 mL) olive oil

1/3 cup (80 mL) balsamic vinegar

3 Tbsp (45 mL) Bragg's (page 10)

3 Tbsp (45 mL) maple syrup

1 tsp (5 mL) Dijon mustard

1. Combine ingredients in a jar, and shake to blend.

almond apricot dressing

MAKES 1 3/4 CUPS (420 ML)

This surprising and delicious dressing was created by Sharada in a moment of playfulness. It's proved to be one of the most requested dressings.

1. In a blender, combine until smooth.

1/4 cup (60 mL) chopped leeks
3 rounded Tbsp (45–50 mL) almond butter or hazelnut butter (or both)
1 tsp (5 mL) tamari
1 cup (240 mL) olive oil
1/2 cup (120 mL) balsamic vinegar
1 cup (240 mL) minced fresh parsley
1 rounded Tbsp (15–20 mL) apricot jam
1 cup (240 mL) water

basilique dressing

MAKES 2–2 1/2 CUPS (480–600 ML) DEPENDING ON HOW MUCH WATER IS ADDED.

Basil was considered a holy herb in the ancient Mediterranean world.

3 rounded Tbsp (45–50 mL) chopped leeks

3 rounded Tbsp (45–50 mL) tahini

1 cup (240 mL) olive oil

1/2 cup (120 mL) balsamic vinegar

1 tsp (5 mL) tamari

2 tsp (10 mL) honey

1/2 tsp (2 mL) pepper

1 1/2 cups (360 mL) fresh basil

1/2–1 cup (120–240 mL) water

1. In a blender, combine until smooth.

honey-mustard dressing

MAKES 3 CUPS (720 ML)

Use only the best quality Dijon mustard for the best quality dressing.

1. In a blender, combine until smooth.

1/4 cup (60 mL) chopped leeks

1 cup (240 mL) olive oil

1/2 cup (120 mL) balsamic vinegar

4 rounded Tbsp (60–70 mL) tahini

1 Tbsp (15 mL) Dijon mustard

2 Tbsp (30 mL) honey

2 Tbsp (30 mL) tamari

1/2 tsp (2 mL) salt

1/2 tsp (2 mL) pepper

1 cup (240 mL) water

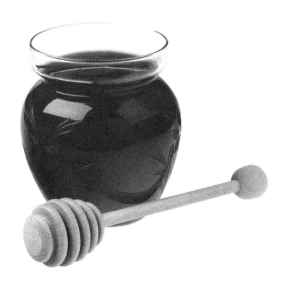

miso-ginger dressing

MAKES 3 CUPS (720 ML)

Ginger and miso have always been good partners, and this dressing proves it.

1/4 cup (60 mL) chopped leeks

1 cup (240 mL) olive oil

1/2 cup (120 mL) balsamic vinegar

1 rounded Tbsp (15–20 mL) grated
   fresh ginger

4 rounded Tbsp (60–70 mL) miso

1 tsp (5 mL) honey

1 rounded Tbsp (15–20 mL) tahini

1 cup (240 mL) water

1. In a blender, combine until smooth.

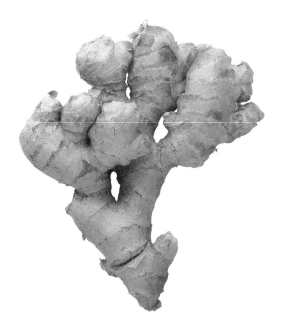

tomato-avocado dressing

MAKES 4 3/4 CUPS (1.14 L)

Rich, thick, creamy—a lovely way to serve fresh greens.

1. In a blender, combine until smooth.

3 cups (720 mL) chopped Roma
tomatoes (about 7)
1 large avocado
1 2/3 cups (400 mL) olive oil
2/3 cup (160 mL) balsamic vinegar
1 cup (240 mL) chopped leeks
1/2 tsp (2 mL) salt
1/2 tsp (2 mL) pepper
5 Tbsp (75 mL) basil

avocado-tomato dressing

MAKES 3 CUPS (720 ML)

Variation on a theme, this time with lemon and dillweed.

4 rounded Tbsp (60–70 mL) chopped
   leeks

1 large avocado

1 cup (240 mL) chopped tomatoes

1 cup (240 mL) olive oil

1/8–1/4 cup (30–60 mL) fresh lemon
   juice (depending on your fondness
   for lemon)

1/3 cup (80 mL) balsamic vinegar

1 Tbsp (15 mL) honey

1 Tbsp (15 mL) dillweed

1 cup (240 mL) water

1. In a blender, combine until smooth.

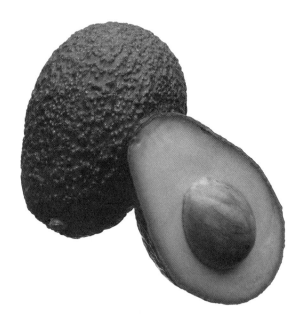

tomato-yogurt dressing

MAKES 3 2/3 CUPS (880 ML)

Fresh tomatoes and herbs. A pretty, soft pink dressing that works well over cold pasta and rice as well.

1. In a blender, combine until smooth.

1 1/2 cups (360 mL) yogurt

2 cups (480 mL) chopped tomatoes

1/3 cup (80 mL) chopped leeks

1/2 cup (120 mL) minced fresh
   parsley

1/3 cup (80 mL) minced fresh
   dillweed

5 Tbsp (75 mL) olive oil

1/4 cup (60 mL) balsamic vinegar

1 Tbsp (15 mL) honey

2 Tbsp (30 mL) tamari

1/2 tsp (2 mL) pepper

parsley-dill dressing

Parsley and dill are a great combination.

3 Tbsp (45 mL) chopped leeks

3 rounded Tbsp (45–50 mL) tahini

1 cup (240 mL) olive oil

1/2 cup (120 mL) balsamic vinegar

1/2 cup (120 mL) minced fresh
  parsley

1/2 cup (120 mL) minced fresh
  dillweed

1 tsp (5 mL) tamari

1/2 tsp (2 mL) salt

1/2 tsp (2 mL) pepper

1 tsp (5 mL) honey

1 cup (240 mL) water

1. In a blender, combine until smooth.

yogurt-dill dressing

The special ingredient of this salad dressing is the fresh dillweed. Use low-fat yogurt for calorie consciousness.

1. In a blender, combine until smooth.

2 cups (480 mL) yogurt
1 cup (240 mL) olive oil
1/4 cup (60 mL) balsamic vinegar
1/3 cup (80 mL) chopped leeks
1 Tbsp (15 mL) tamari
1/2 tsp (2 mL) salt
1/2 tsp (2 mL) pepper
2–3 rounded Tbsp (30–50 mL) honey
1 cup (240 mL) fresh dillweed

yogurt-parsley dressing

MAKES 2 1/2 CUPS (600 ML)

Lemon adds a nice citrus touch to this dressing. You can use low-fat yogurt.

1 3/4 cups (420 mL) yogurt

1/3 cup (80 mL) olive oil

1/3 cup (80 mL) chopped leeks

1/4 cup (60 mL) fresh lemon juice

1 cup (240 mL) minced fresh parsley

1 Tbsp (15 mL) tamari

1/2 tsp (2 mL) salt

1/2 tsp (2 mL) pepper

3 Tbsp (45 mL) maple syrup

1. In a blender, combine until smooth.

vasudev's unorthodox chutney

MAKES 3 1/2 CUPS (840 ML)

It works! A great chutney that resulted from a stream-of-consciousness approach to cooking.

1. Combine all the ingredients in a saucepan, and simmer until the water is absorbed and the flavours are well blended.

1 1/2 cups (360 mL) chopped dates

3/4 cup (180 mL) currants

2 medium apples, peeled, cored, and chopped

1/4 cup (60 mL) orange juice

2 Tbsp (30 mL) finely minced or grated ginger

1/2 cup (120 mL) Sucanat or turbinado sugar

1/2 cup (120 mL) apple cider vinegar

1/4 cup (60 mL) rice milk

1 cup (240 mL) water

1 1/2–2 tsp (7–10 mL) cinnamon

1 tsp (5 mL) cardamom

1/2 tsp (2 mL) nutmeg

Pinch cloves

1 cup (240 mL) grated coconut

TIPS CHUTNEY

• Keeps in the fridge for at least a week.

ramanand's apple chutney

MAKES 2 CUPS (480 ML)

A more traditional approach to chutney by Ramanand, one of our cooks who makes great Indian food. A must-have with any curry dish.

3 medium apples, peeled, cored, and chopped

1/3 cup (80 mL) finely minced leeks

1/3 cup (80 mL) turbinado sugar or Sucanat

3/4 tsp (3 mL) grated or finely minced ginger

1 cup (240 mL) apple cider vinegar

1/3 cup (80 mL) currants

1/2 tsp (2 mL) salt

1 tsp (5 mL) chili powder

1/2 heaping tsp (2 mL) curry powder

1 heaping tsp (5 mL) garam masala

1. In a saucepan, combine all the ingredients except the garam masala, and simmer until the apples are soft.

2. Add the garam masala when the apples begin to get soft and cook a few minutes more.

TIPS   **CHUTNEY**

• Keeps in the fridge for at least a week.

eggplant relish

Nice crispy texture. More pungent with balsamic vinegar, milder with the vinegar combo. A unique condiment for burgers and savoury loaves.

1. Place the peeled and cubed eggplant in a colander, and generously sprinkle salt over it. Set it aside for 10 to 15 minutes.
2. Rinse the eggplant under cold water, then steam it until it's soft. Remove from the heat and let it cool.
3. Blend the eggplant in a food processor.
4. Combine the eggplant and all the other ingredients in a mixing bowl.
5. It's best refrigerated overnight before serving.

1 medium eggplant, peeled and cubed
Salt
2 1/2–3 cups (600–720 mL) chopped celery
1 1/2–2 cups (360–480 mL) chopped green pepper
1–1 1/2 cups (240–360 mL) chopped red pepper
1 1/2–2 cups (360–380 mL) chopped leeks
1/2 cup (120 mL) balsamic vinegar (or 1/4 cup [60 mL] apple cider vinegar and 1/4 cup [60 mL] balsamic vinegar)
1/2 tsp (2 mL) salt
1/4–1/2 tsp (1–2 mL) pepper
1/4 cup (60 mL) turbinado sugar

TIPS   RELISH

• Keeps in the fridge for at least a week.

salsa

MAKES 5 CUPS (1.2 L)

Piquant and easy to make. Your tortilla chips will cry out for this salsa!

3 cups (720 mL) finely minced
  tomatoes
2 cups (480 mL) finely minced
  green peppers
1/4 cup (60 mL) finely minced leeks
3 Tbsp (45 mL) fresh lemon juice
3 Tbsp (45 mL) juice from pickled
  jalapenos
1 tsp (5 mL) salt
2–2 1/2 finely minced pickled
  jalapenos or 1 finely minced fresh
  jalapeno
1 medium avocado, mashed

1. Mix all the ingredients in a bowl. Refrigerate and allow the mixture to marinate for a few hours (or overnight) before serving.

tahini-ginger **sauce**

MAKES 4 1/2 CUPS (1.08 L)

Spicy and stunningly delicious. Once you try this sauce, it will become one of your favourites—guaranteed! Try it served over grains or vegetables or Martha's Nut Loaf (page 27).

1. Combine the tahini and water in a blender.
2. In a saucepan, combine the leeks, ginger, and the tahini-water mixture. Simmer for 25 to 30 minutes, stirring frequently.
3. Remove the saucepan from the heat, and add the milk or soymilk, lemon juice, tamari, balsamic vinegar, and pepper.
4. Blend the mixture in a food processor or blender until it's smooth.

3/4 cup (180 mL) tahini

1 cup (240 mL) water

1 cup (240 mL) finely minced leeks

1/2 cup (120 mL) finely minced or
grated ginger

1 1/2 cups (360 mL) milk or soymilk

4 1/2 Tbsp (67 mL) fresh lemon
juice

3 Tbsp (45 mL) tamari

1 Tbsp (15 mL) balsamic vinegar

1/4 tsp (1 mL) pepper

tahini-miso sauce

MAKES 4 CUPS (960 ML)

A sauce that will win you accolades when served over grain and vegetables
or any savoury meal.

1 cup (240 mL) finely minced leeks

1/4 cup (60 mL) grated ginger

2 Tbsp (30 mL) olive oil

3/4 cup (180 mL) tahini

2 cups (480 mL) water

4 1/2 Tbsp (67 mL) fresh
   lemon juice

1 cup (240 mL) milk or soymilk

1/2 cup (120 mL) miso

1. In a saucepan, sauté the leeks and ginger in olive oil.
2. Combine the tahini, water, lemon juice, and milk or
soymilk in a blender, then add to the saucepan with
the leek and ginger mixture, and stir.
3. Turn off the heat, and mix the miso in.

mel's sundried tomato and fresh basil pesto

SERVES 4

The name says it all—a taste of summer served over your favourite pasta. Ahhh!

1. Soak the sundried tomatoes in boiling water for about 15 minutes or until they're softened. Reserve the water.

2. Slowly roast the nuts either in the oven or in a frying pan on the stove over low heat. Watch them carefully so they don't burn.

3. In a food processor, grind the roasted nuts and then add the rest of the ingredients. Blend until the mixture is smooth and creamy. If the mixture is too thick, add a bit of the tomato water.

1/2 cup (120 mL) sundried tomatoes

3/4 cup (180 mL) pine nuts or
   cashew nuts

2 cups (480 mL) fresh basil (packed)

1/3 cup (80 mL) olive oil

1/2 tsp (2 mL) salt

1/2 tsp (2 mL) pepper

1/4–1/3 cup (60–80 mL) parmesan
   (dairy or soy)

eggless egg spread

If you didn't know better, you'd swear it had egg in it! Great as a sandwich spread, and it's high in protein.

4 cups (960 mL) mashed tofu

1/2 cup (120 mL) finely minced celery

1/2 cup (120 mL) finely minced leeks

1/2 cup (120 mL) finely minced fresh parsley

1–2 Tbsp (15–30 mL) eggless mayonnaise

2 Tbsp (30 mL) tamari

2 Tbsp (30 mL) Dijon mustard

1 tsp (5 mL) turmeric

1. Mix all the ingredients together, et voilà!

ginger-curry spread

MAKES 2 CUPS (480 ML)

An unusual and zestful spread. With the addition of a little water, it makes a great vegetable dip.

1. Blend all the ingredients in a food processor.

1/3 cup (80 mL) finely minced leeks
1–1 1/2 Tbsp (15–22 mL) finely
   grated ginger
2 cups (480 mL) crumbled tofu
4 Tbsp (60 mL) balsamic vinegar
4 Tbsp (60 mL) olive oil
3 Tbsp (45 mL) tamari
1 Tbsp (15 mL) lemon juice
1 Tbsp (15 mL) chili powder
1 Tbsp (15 mL) curry powder
1/2 tsp (2 mL) salt
Pinch cayenne

TIPS   GINGER

• You can use less ginger if this is too strong for your taste.

sunseed spread

MAKES ABOUT 3 1/2 CUPS (840 ML)

Back by popular demand. From our first cookbook, *Salt Spring Island Cooking,* this is the most frequently requested recipe. Great on bread or crackers.

2 cups (480 mL) sunflower seeds

3 Tbsp (45 mL) olive oil

1/3 cup (80 mL) finely minced leeks

1 lb (454 g) tofu

1/3 cup (80 mL) engevita yeast

5 Tbsp (75 mL) tamari

1/2 tsp (2 mL) pepper

1. Using a food processor, grind the sunflower seeds first, until they're quite fine. Then add the rest of the ingredients and blend until all the ingredients are well mixed.

TIPS   BLENDING

• This recipe can also work in a blender, but you have to add the ingredients one at a time, in the order listed, and you might need a bit of water to help with the blending.

mushroom-feta topping

Why not try this on toast or as a complement to any grain or savoury loaf?

1. Sauté the leeks in olive oil until they become soft.
2. Add the mushrooms and tamari. Sauté briefly, then add the tomatoes, parsley, and pepper. Cover the pan and simmer until the tomatoes are cooked in.
3. Add the feta and mix it in. Cook very briefly and serve hot.

2 Tbsp (30 mL) olive oil

1 cup (240 mL) chopped leeks

5 cups (1.2 L) chopped mushrooms

1 Tbsp (15 mL) tamari

1 cup (240 mL) chopped tomatoes

1/2 cup (120 mL) minced fresh parsley

1/4–1/2 tsp (1–2 mL) pepper

1 cup (240 mL) crumbled or grated feta

ann's jalapeno cornbread

SERVES 8–10

A cornbread bursting with flavour.

1/2 cup (120 mL) cornmeal

1/2 cup (120 mL) polenta
(corn grits)

1/2 cup (120 mL) flour

2 Tbsp (30 mL) baking powder

1/2 tsp (2 mL) salt

1 cup (240 mL) finely minced leeks

1/2 tsp (2 mL) chili flakes (optional)

4-oz tin (112 g) chopped green
chilies

1 cup (240 mL) grated cheese
(cheddar or soy)

2 tsp (10 mL) blackstrap molasses

1 1/2 tsp (7 mL) egg replacer mixed
with 1 Tbsp (15 mL) of water

1 cup (240 mL) milk or soymilk

1. Mix dry ingredients together in a large mixing bowl, then add the rest of the ingredients.
2. Transfer the batter into a greased 8 x 8 inch (20 x 20 cm) baking pan.
3. Bake at 375°F (190°C) for 40 minutes or until the top is brown and crisp.

TIPS WHEAT-FREE

• To make this cornbread wheat-free, replace the wheat flour with brown rice flour and add one tablespoon ground flaxseed that has been soaked in one tablespoon of hot water for 15 minutes.

donna's focaccia

MAKES 1 ROUND FLAT LOAF

Impress your guests by making focaccia bread in the traditional Italian way.

1. In a large mixing bowl, dissolve the yeast in warm water. Let it stand until the yeast is softened (about 5 minutes).
2. Stir in the salt and oil.
3. Gradually mix in 3 cups of flour to make a soft dough. Use more flour if necessary. You may need up to 4 cups.
4. Turn the dough onto a floured surface, and knead it until it's smooth and elastic. Add more flour as needed.
5. Turn the dough over in a greased bowl. Cover the bowl and let the dough rise in a warm place until it's doubled in size (about an hour).
6. Punch the dough down. Then turn it out again onto a lightly floured surface. With a floured rolling pin, roll the dough into a half-inch thick round.
7. Place the round dough on a lightly floured baking sheet. Make slight fingertip indentations over the top of the focaccia.
8. For the topping, spread the olive oil over the bread dough. Sprinkle with the herbs and then the parmesan.
9. Bake at 400°F (205°C) for 15 to 20 minutes or until the bottom crust is lightly browned.

Crust:

1 Tbsp (15 mL) dry yeast

1 cup (240 mL) warm water

1/2 tsp (2 mL) salt

2 tsp (10 mL) olive oil

3–4 cups (720–960 mL) unbleached white flour (or 1/2 whole wheat and 1/2 unbleached white)

Topping:

2–3 Tbsp (30–45 mL) olive oil

1 Tbsp (15 mL) basil

1 Tbsp (15 mL) rosemary

3 Tbsp (45 mL) parmesan cheese

krista's banana-ginger bread

Banana bread with a difference. Try it for breakfast or with an afternoon cup of tea.

3 medium bananas

Juice of 1 medium lemon

1/4 cup (60 mL) oil or butter

1 Tbsp (15 mL) blackstrap molasses

1/4 cup (60 mL) milk or soymilk

1/2 cup (120 mL) turbinado sugar

3 Tbsp (45 mL) minced fresh ginger

1 Tbsp (15 mL) grated lemon rind

1 1/2 cups (360 mL) whole wheat
pastry flour (or spelt)

1/2 cup (120 mL) brown rice flour

1/2 tsp (2 mL) baking powder

1/2 tsp (2 mL) baking soda

1/2 tsp (2 mL) salt

1/2 cup (120 mL) grated coconut

1. Combine the wet ingredients in a mixing bowl. Mix in the sugar and ginger.
2. In a separate bowl, combine the dry ingredients.
3. Fold the wet and dry ingredients together.
4. Pour the batter into a greased 5 1/2 x 9 1/2 inch (approx. 13 1/2 x 24 cm) bread pan.
5. Bake at 350°F (180°C) for 45 minutes.

TIPS   WHEAT-FREE

• To make this bread wheat-free, replace the wheat flour with brown rice flour. Soak 4 tablespoons (60 mL) of ground flaxseed in 1/4 cup (60 mL) hot water for 15 minutes, and add to the wet ingredients.

KRISTA, A RESIDENT IN OUR COMMUNITY for several months and the joyful tester of many muffin and quickbread recipes, offered to contribute her favourite banana bread recipe. She had it written somewhere, but since it didn't seem to want to be found, she tried it from memory. It took a few tries before she was satisfied. Although we enthusiastically ate all the rejects, we had to admit this was the best. After all the testing was done, she found the recipe, only to discover she had replicated it perfectly.

mel's irish soda bread

MAKES TWO BEAUTIFUL ROUND, LIGHT LOAVES.

Mel, who lived in our community with her family for a couple of years, prepared numerous delicious dishes, including this ever-popular bread.

1. Mix all the dry ingredients together in a mixing bowl. Cut the butter into the flour mixture.
2. When the flour and butter are well blended, add the buttermilk or soured soymilk and mix it in. The dough will be a bit sticky, but you should be able to shape it into a ball.
3. Cut the dough into 2 equal portions and shape each one into a ball. Form them into round loaves about 2 inches (5 cm) high.
4. Using a buttered chopstick, make a cross on top of each loaf. Don't cut into the loaf, but rather indent by pushing the chopstick down.
5. Place the loaves on a buttered cookie sheet, leaving 3 to 4 inches (8 to 10 cm) between them.
6. If you want a crunchy crust, sprinkle a bit of sugar on the top of the loaves.
7. Bake at 350°F (180°C) for 40 to 45 minutes or until the loaves are golden brown. To check if the bread is ready, insert a knife into the middle of the loaf. If it comes out clean, the bread is done.

7 cups (1.68 L) unbleached white flour

2 tsp (10 mL) salt

1 heaping Tbsp (15–20 mL) baking soda

1/2–2/3 cup (120–160 mL) turbinado sugar

1 heaping Tbsp (15–20 mL) cream of tartar

5 Tbsp (75 mL) butter

3 1/4 cups (780 mL) buttermilk (or milk or soymilk soured with 2 Tbsp [30 mL] vinegar or lemon juice)

banana-yogurt muffins

MAKES 1 DOZEN

Delicious and nutritious at the same time.

1 1/2 cups (360 mL) whole wheat
   pastry or spelt flour

1 cup (240 mL) 100% bran cereal or
   natural bran

1 tsp (5 mL) baking powder

1 tsp (5 mL) baking soda

1/2 cup (120 mL) turbinado sugar

1/2 cup (120 mL) chopped nuts

1/2 cup (120 mL) raisins

1 1/2 Tbsp (22 mL) ground flaxseed

1 cup (240 mL) mashed banana
   (2 medium bananas)

3/4 cup (180 mL) yogurt

3/4 cup (180 mL) melted butter
   or ghee (page 41)

1. Combine the dry ingredients in a mixing bowl.
2. Combine the wet ingredients in a separate bowl.
3. Fold the wet and dry ingredients together.
4. Fill greased muffin tins with the batter.
5. Bake at 400°F (205°C) for 20 to 25 minutes.

TIPS   WHEAT-FREE

• To make these muffins wheat-free, replace the wheat flour with brown rice flour and the bran cereal or wheat bran with oat bran.

• Also, soak 5 tablespoons of ground flaxseed in 5 tablespoons hot water for 15 minutes, and add to the wet ingredients.

carrot-date muffins

MAKES 1 DOZEN

An unusual combination that's sweetly delicious.

1. Chop the dates, then soak them in boiling water for about 20 minutes or until they're soft. (Soaking time may vary depending on packaging and age of dates.) Discard water.
2. Combine the dry ingredients in a mixing bowl.
3. Mix in the carrots, milk, dates, oil, vinegar, and orange rind in a separate bowl.
4. Fold the wet and dry ingredients together.
5. Spoon the batter into greased muffin tins.
6. Bake at 350°F (180°C) for 20 to 25 minutes.

1/2 cup (120 mL) chopped dates

1/4 cup (60 mL) boiling water

2 cups (480 mL) whole wheat pastry or spelt flour

1/2 cup (120 mL) turbinado sugar

1 tsp (5 mL) salt

1 tsp (5 mL) baking soda

1 tsp (5 mL) baking powder

1 cup (240 mL) grated carrots

1 cup (240 mL) milk, soymilk, or rice milk

1/4 cup (60 mL) vegetable oil

1 Tbsp (15 mL) cider vinegar

1 Tbsp (15 mL) grated orange rind

TIPS WHEAT-FREE

• To make these muffins wheat-free, replace the wheat flour with brown rice flour.

• Also, soak 4 tablespoons (60 mL) of ground flaxseed in 1/4 cup (60 mL) hot water for 15 minutes, and add to the wet ingredients.

karen's pineapple-banana muffins

MAKES 1 DOZEN

Karen, a mom of children in the Centre school, brought these one day as an after-school snack. The kids weren't the only ones to eat them, and we asked her if we could use the recipe in this book.

3 medium bananas, mashed
  (about 1 1/2 cups [360 mL])
1/2 cup (120 mL) pineapple, drained
  and chopped
1/3 cup (80 mL) vegetable oil
1 1/2 tsp (17 mL) egg replacer
  mixed with 1 Tbsp (15 mL) water
1 cup (240 mL) whole wheat pastry
  or spelt flour
1 tsp (5 mL) baking soda
1 tsp (5 mL) baking powder
3/4 cup (180 mL) turbinado sugar
3 Tbsp (45 mL) grated coconut
1/2 cup (120 mL) whole sunflower
  seeds
1/2 cup (120 mL) natural bran

1. Combine the wet ingredients in a mixing bowl.
2. Combine the dry ingredients in a separate bowl.
3. Fold the wet and dry ingredients together.
4. Spoon the batter into greased muffin tins.
5. Bake at 375°F (190°C) for 20 minutes.

TIPS — WHEAT-FREE

• To make these muffins wheat-free, replace the wheat flour with brown rice flour and the bran with oatbran.
• Also, soak 4 tablespoons (60 mL) of ground flaxseed in 1/4 cup (60 mL) hot water for 15 minutes, and add to the wet ingredients.

orange-date muffins

MAKES 1 DOZEN

One of the happiest taste combinations.

1. Soak the dates in the boiling water until they're softened. Purée 3/4 of the dates with the water used for soaking them.
2. Chop the remaining dates into chunks.
3. Mix the date purée and date chunks with the rest of the wet ingredients in a mixing bowl.
4. Mix the dry ingredients in a separate mixing bowl.
5. Fold the wet and dry ingredients together.
6. Fill greased muffin tins with the batter.
7. Bake at 350°F (180°C) for 20 to 25 minutes.

1 3/4 cups (420 mL) dates
1 1/4 cups (300 mL) boiling water
Grated rind of 2 oranges
Juice of 2 oranges (about 6 oz [168 g])
1 Tbsp (15 mL) vinegar
1 tsp (5 mL) vanilla extract
1/4 cup (60 mL) vegetable oil
1/4 cup (60 mL) soymilk
2 cups (480 mL) whole wheat pastry or spelt flour
1 tsp (5 mL) baking powder
1 tsp (5 mL) baking soda
1 tsp (5 mL) salt
1/2 cup (120 mL) turbinado sugar
1/2 cup (120 mL) ground almonds

TIPS   WHEAT-FREE

• To make these muffins wheat-free, replace the wheat flour with brown rice flour.
• Also, soak 4 tablespoons (60 mL) of ground flaxseed in 1/4 cup (60 mL) hot water for 15 minutes, and add to the wet ingredients.

zucchini muffins

MAKES 1 DOZEN

A moist and delicious solution to zucchini overload.

1/2 cup (120 mL) raisins

1/2 cup (120 mL) boiling water

2 cups (480 mL) flour (whole wheat
  pastry or spelt)

1 cup (240 mL) turbinado sugar

1 1/2 tsp (7 mL) baking powder

1 1/2 tsp (7 mL) baking soda

1 Tbsp (15 mL) cinnamon

1 tsp (5 mL) salt

1 cup (240 mL) grated raw zucchini

1/2 cup (120 mL) milk or soymilk

1/4 cup (60 mL) vegetable oil

1 Tbsp (15 mL) cider vinegar

1 tsp (5 mL) vanilla extract

1. Soak the raisins in boiling water until they're soft.
2. In a bowl, mix all the dry ingredients together.
3. Mix the wet ingredients, including the raisins and water, in another bowl.
4. Combine the wet and dry ingredients.
5. Grease and flour a muffin tin and fill the muffin cups with the batter.
6. Bake at 350°F (180°C) for 20 to 25 minutes.

TIPS   WHEAT-FREE

• To make these muffins wheat-free, replace the wheat flour with brown rice flour.

• Also, soak 4 tablespoons (60 mL) of ground flaxseed in 1/4 cup (60 mL) hot water for 15 minutes, and add to the wet ingredients.

almond cookies

MAKES 2 DOZEN COOKIES

Crispy lunchbox cookies. Betcha can't eat just one!

1. Grind the almonds until they're fine.
2. Cream the butter and sugar.
3. Add the salt and almond or vanilla extract to the butter-sugar mixture.
4. Mix the dry ingredients together, including the ground almonds.
5. Mix the wet and dry ingredients together.
6. Chill the dough for half an hour, until it's firm enough to handle.
7. Roll the dough into small balls and press them onto an oiled cookie sheet.
8. Bake at 325°F (165°C) for 25 to 30 minutes.

1/2 cup (120 mL) almonds

1 cup (240 mL) butter

3/4 cup (180 mL) turbinado sugar

1/8 tsp (1/2 mL) salt

3 tsp (15 mL) almond extract or vanilla extract

1 cup (240 mL) whole wheat pastry flour

1 cup (240 mL) brown rice flour

TIPS — WHEAT-FREE

- You can make these cookies wheat-free by using all brown rice flour.
- Also, soak 4 tablespoons (60 mL) ground flaxseeds in 1/4 cup (60 mL) hot water for 15 minutes and add to the wet ingredients.

mary's almond pie crust

Winner of the "Best Tasting Pie Crust" for 2001 on Salt Spring Island (or would be if there were such a contest). It may be tricky to get into the pie plate because there is no gluten in rice flour, but it's worth it!

1 cup (240 mL) brown rice flour

3/4 cup (180 mL) whole wheat pastry flour

2/3 cup (160 mL) turbinado sugar

2/3 cup (160 mL) butter

1/2 cup (120 mL) finely ground almonds

1/4 cup (60 mL) cold water

1. Combine the flours and sugar. Add the butter, and either mix it in a food processor or cut it in with a pastry cutter until the mixture is crumbly.

2. If you're using a food processor, this is the time to remove the mixture and place it in a mixing bowl.

3. Add the ground almonds and knead them into the crust.

4. Add the cold water, and knead the dough until it forms a soft ball.

5. Flour a board and roll out the dough on it. Lift the dough with spatulas and place it into a greased pie pan, pressing the dough into the pan.

6. Pre-bake the crust at 350°F (180°C) for 10 to 12 minutes, then remove it from the oven and pour the pie filling into it.

7. Baking times and temperature will vary for the different pies, so follow the directions for the recipe you're using.

TIPS
WHEAT-FREE

• To make this pie crust wheat-free, use all brown rice flour.

• Also, soak 4 tablespoons (60 mL) ground flaxseeds in 1/4 cup (60 mL) hot water for 15 minutes, and add it to the dough instead of 1/4 cup cold water.

apple crumble

SERVES 12

Although myth has it that Eve tempted Adam with an apple, women's wisdom shows it was actually a piece of apple crumble.

1. To make the crumble, cream the butter and sugar. Add the flour, oats, and cinnamon and mix together.
2. Pat two-thirds of the mixture into the bottom of a 9 x 11 inch baking pan (23 x 26 cm).
3. In a mixing bowl, mix the sliced apples, sugar, cinnamon, and butter.
4. Place it on top of the bottom crust in the baking pan.
5. Spread the remaining crumble mixture over the top and pat it down.
6. Bake at 350°F (180°C) for 55 minutes to one hour.

Crumble:
1 1/2 cups (360 mL) butter
1 1/2 cups (360 mL) turbinado sugar
2 cups (480 mL) whole wheat pastry
  or spelt flour
4 cups (960 mL) oats
1 Tbsp (15 mL) cinnamon

Filling:
12 cups (2.9 L) thinly sliced apples
  (about 12 medium)
1/2 cup (120 mL) turbinado sugar
1 1/2 Tbsp (22 mL) cinnamon
1/4 cup (60 mL) butter

TIPS
VERY BERRY

• A berry crumble is a delicious alternative—try blueberries, raspberries, blackberries—your choice. You'll need a thickener to hold the berries together, so add 2 tablespoons (30 mL) arrowroot powder mixed in 1/2 cup (120 mL) water to the filling.

TIPS
WHEAT-FREE

• To make this crumble wheat-free, use all oats instead of oats and flour—or replace the wheat flour with rice flour.

apple strudel

Looks very professional and tastes as good as it looks. Not difficult to make at all. Eat it while it's still warm for the best crispy texture.

3 cups (720 mL) thinly sliced apples
  (about 4 medium)

2 Tbsp (30 mL) arrowroot powder

1/4 cup (60 mL) orange juice

1 Tbsp (15 mL) fresh lemon juice

1/2 cup (120 mL) toasted nuts
  (almonds, walnuts, or pecans)

1/4 cup (60 mL) raisins

1/3 cup (80 mL) turbinado sugar

1 Tbsp (15 mL) cinnamon

1 tsp (5 mL) nutmeg

24 sheets filo pastry

1/3–1/2 cup (80–120 mL) melted
  butter or ghee (page 00)

1. Place the sliced apples in a mixing bowl, and sprinkle them with arrowroot powder.
2. Add the orange juice and lemon juice and mix in.
3. Add the nuts, raisins, sugar, cinnamon, and nutmeg and mix in.
4. On a dry surface, lay one sheet of filo pastry, and brush it with melted butter or ghee. Cover it with a second sheet of filo and brush it with butter. Repeat this process two more times for a total of 4 sheets of filo.
5. Place about 3/4 cup (180 mL) of the apple mixture in the centre of the filo, and spread it out in a line across the width of the filo, leaving a bit of space at each edge.
6. Fold the filo over the filling, bringing the edges of the filo together.
7. Fold the sides in toward the centre.
8. Roll it up, and place it with the edge side down on a greased baking sheet.
9. Do the same for each roll.
10. Brush the tops of all the rolls with melted butter or ghee.
11. Bake at 350°F (180°C) for 15 to 20 minutes until the filo is golden brown and crisp.

5

6

fold   fold
7

apple-yogurt cake

SERVES 8–10

A moist, delicate cake to serve with afternoon tea.

1. Mix the dry ingredients in a mixing bowl.
2. Mix the rest of the ingredients in a separate bowl.
3. Combine the dry ingredients with the wet ingredients in one bowl.
4. Spoon the batter into a greased 8 x 8 inch (20 x 20 cm) baking pan.
5. Bake at 350°F (180°C) for 40 to 45 minutes or until a toothpick inserted into the middle comes out clean.

1 1/2 cups (360 mL) flour (whole wheat pastry or spelt)
1 cup (240 mL) turbinado sugar
1 tsp (5 mL) baking soda
1 tsp (5 mL) cinnamon
1 tsp (5 mL) ground cardamom
1/2 tsp (2 mL) ground ginger powder
1/2 tsp (2 mL) salt
2 tsp (10 mL) grated orange rind
1 1/2 cups (360 mL) yogurt
1 Tbsp (15 mL) arrowroot powder dissolved in 1/4 cup (60 mL) milk, rice milk, or soymilk
1 1/2 cups (360 mL) coarsely chopped or grated apple
2–3 tsp (10–15 mL) vanilla extract

TIPS WHEAT-FREE

- To make this cake wheat-free, replace the wheat flour with brown rice flour.
- Also, replace the arrowroot powder and water with 4 tablespoons (60 mL) ground flaxseed soaked for 15 minutes in 1/4 cup (60 mL) hot water.

sharada's banana coconut cream pie

Yes, we did it—a cream pie without cream and eggs! Better than the original. Sharada left the test pie in the fridge to set, and when she came back an hour later it was almost all gone! Try this with the almond pie crust (page 104).

2 medium bananas (about 1 cup [240 mL] mashed)

2 13.5-oz tins (800 mL) coconut milk

1/3 cup (80 mL) arrowroot powder

1/3 cup (80 mL) water

1/4 cup (60 mL) turbinado sugar

2 tsp (10 mL) vanilla extract

1/4 cup (60 mL) grated coconut

1. Blend the banana in a food processor, then add the coconut milk and blend them together.

2. Mix the arrowroot powder with the water, and add it to the banana mixture.

3. Add all the remaining ingredients except the coconut.

4. Blend until smooth.

5. Pour the mixture into a saucepan and cook it over medium-low heat until it begins to boil and thicken, stirring it constantly with a whisk.

6. Remove the saucepan from the heat and allow it to cool a bit before pouring it into a pre-baked pie shell.

7. Toast the coconut in a pan over medium-low heat until it begins to brown. Keep stirring it so that it doesn't burn.

8. Allow it to cool enough to handle. Then sprinkle it over the pie.

9. Chill the pie before serving.

banana-date topping

MAKES ENOUGH TO COVER 1 CAKE

Asia, at age ten, has all the predilections of a great cook. It was she who adjusted the flavours for this topping. Try the results yourself—fabulous! And watch for Asia's own cookbook (in about 15 years).

1. Soak the dates in the boiling water until they're soft.
2. Blend the dates and water in a food processor until the mixture is smooth.
3. Add the bananas, and blend until smooth.
4. Add the remaining ingredients and blend again.
5. Spread over a cooled cake.

2 cups (480 mL) pitted dates

1 cup (240 mL) boiling water

2 medium bananas (about 1 cup [240 mL] mashed)

Juice of 2 lemons

4 cups (960 mL) milk or soymilk

2 tsp (10 mL) cinnamon

1/2 tsp (2 mL) nutmeg

bliss balls

Best alternative to a Power Bar—pop one in your mouth and get going!

1/2 cup (120 mL) almonds
1/2 cup (120 mL) raisins
1/2 cup (120 mL) tahini
1/4 cup (60 mL) honey
2 tsp (10 mL) cinnamon
2 tsp (10 mL) cardamom
1/2 cup (120 mL) chocolate chips
1/3 cup (80 mL) grated coconut

1. Grind the almonds fine in a food processor.
2. Add the raisins and grind until they're chopped up.
3. Add the tahini, honey, cinnamon, and cardamom, and blend until everything is well mixed.
4. Empty the mixture into a mixing bowl, and hand-mix the chocolate chips in.
5. Put the coconut into a shallow bowl or a plate.
6. Form balls from the mixture, roll them in the coconut, and arrange them on a platter.
7. Keep them refrigerated.

cheesecake

SERVES 6–8

The real thing! Salt Spring's answer to New York's famous recipe. Top with a sweet sauce, such as Raspberry-Blueberry Sauce (page 131).

Filling:
1. In a saucepan, heat the sugar and milk or rice milk over low heat until the sugar is dissolved.
2. Let the milk and sugar mixture cool.
3. Blend all the ingredients together in a food processor until it's smooth.

Crust:
1. Cream the butter with the sugar and graham cracker, then mix in the remaining ingredients.
2. Press into the bottom of a pie plate (a spring-form pan is best).

Assembly:
1. Pour the filling on top of the crust.
2. Bake at 300°F (140°C) for 40 minutes or until the filling is set and beginning to brown.
3. Allow it to cool, then spread a sauce (Raspberry-Blueberry Sauce [page 131] or your preference) over the cheesecake.
4. Refrigerate before serving.

Filling:
1 cup (240 mL) turbinado sugar
1/8 cup (30 mL) milk or rice milk
3 cups (720 mL) cream cheese
1 1/2 cups (360 mL) yogurt
1 1/2 tsp (7 mL) vanilla extract
1 Tbsp (15 mL) arrowroot powder

Crust:
3/4 cup (180 mL) butter
2 Tbsp (30 mL) turbinado sugar
1 1/2 cups (360 mL) graham cracker crumbs
6 Tbsp (90 mL) ground rolled oats
6 Tbsp (90 mL) ground walnuts
1 tsp (5 mL) cinnamon
1/4 tsp (1 mL) nutmeg

TIPS — WHEAT-FREE

- You can make this cheesecake wheat-free by replacing the graham cracker crumbs with 1 1/4 cups (300 mL) coarsely ground oats and 1 cup (240 mL) ground walnuts.

vasudev's fruit compote

SERVES 6

Delicious served with yogurt.

3 medium apples

2 medium pears

1 medium orange

Juice of 1/2 lemon

1/2 cup (120 mL) dates, pitted and
   chopped

3/4 cup (180 mL) currants
   or 1/2 cup (120 mL) raisins

1 cup (240 mL) water

2 tsp (10 mL) cinnamon

1/2 tsp (2 mL) cardamom

1/4 tsp (1 mL) allspice

1/4 tsp (1 mL) nutmeg

1 tsp (5 mL) finely grated lemon
   peel (optional)

1. Peel, core, and cube the apples and pears.

2. Peel the orange and cut it into small pieces.

3. Combine all the ingredients in a pot and stir frequently over medium-low heat.

4. Keep an eye on the thickness. If it's getting thick, but the fruit is not yet soft, add another 1/4 to 1/2 cup (60–120 mL) water.

linda's date squares

Linda has graciously shared her recipe for these sweet and delicious date squares.

1. In a saucepan, cook the dates and water until the dates are soft.
2. Add the orange juice and lemon juice, and cook until most of the liquid is absorbed.
3. To make the crust, cream the butter and sugar.
4. Add the dry ingredients and mix well, either by hand or in a food processor.
5. To assemble, pat two-thirds of the crust mixture into the bottom of a greased 11 x 15 inch (24 x 42.5 cm) pan.
6. Using a spatula, spread the date filling evenly over the crust.
7. Press the remaining crust mixture on top of the dates.
8. Bake at 350°F (180°C) for 35 to 40 minutes or until lightly browned.

Filling:

1 lb (454 g) chopped dates

1 cup (240 mL) water

1/4 cup (60 mL) orange juice

3 Tbsp (45 mL) fresh lemon juice

Crust:

1 1/2 cups (360 mL) butter

1 1/2 cups (360 mL) turbinado sugar

3 cups (720 mL) oats

3 cups (720 mL) flour (whole wheat pastry or spelt)

1 tsp (5 mL) baking soda

2 tsp (10 mL) baking powder

1/2 tsp (2 mL) salt

THESE DAYS YOU'RE MORE LIKELY TO SEE LINDA in a kayak on the ocean, but not too long ago she ran a popular health food store/restaurant on Salt Spring Island. The food was great, the atmosphere warm and relaxing. Many of us were sad to see Linda's place close—now there's no comparable place on Salt Spring to go for a gourmet vegetarian meal (except, of course, the Salt Spring Centre). Thanks, Linda, for sharing this recipe with us.

TIPS
WHEAT-FREE

• You can make these date squares wheat-free by using all oats instead of oats and flour.

mark's accidental peanut butter cookies

MAKES 1 1/2–2 DOZEN COOKIES (DEPENDING ON SIZE)

These cookies are the results of Salt Spring Centre School teacher Mark's first culinary adventure. Here is the astonishingly delicious result. Bravo Mark!

3/4 cup (180 mL) turbinado sugar

1/3 cup (80 mL) butter

1 3/4 cups (420 mL) flour

3/4 cup (180 mL) peanut butter

2 Tbsp (30 mL) milk, soymilk, or rice milk

1 tsp (5 mL) vanilla extract

1 tsp (5 mL) baking soda

1/2 tsp (2 mL) salt

1. Cream the butter and sugar, then add the rest of the ingredients and mix well, either with a food processor or by hand in a bowl.

2. Roll the batter into small balls, place them on an ungreased cookie sheet, and flatten them with a fork.

3. Bake at 375°F (190°C) for 10 to 15 minutes.

mayana's gran's carrot pudding

MAKES 2 PUDDINGS, EACH SERVING 6-8

A family recipe dating back to the 1870s, and made every Christmas since—but you don't have to wait for Christmas to try it. Traditionally served with Lemon Sauce. Try either version on pages 129 and 130.

1. In a small bowl, mix together the flour, baking powder, and spices.

2. In a large mixing bowl, combine together all of the remaining ingredients in the given order.

3. Add the dry ingredients to the wet ingredients and mix well.

4. Divide the mixture evenly and press into two greased pudding bowls. (You can use any kind of bowl as long as it can be steamed. Ceramic or Pyrex would be fine, but not something that might crack.)

5. Cover the bowls with waxed or brown paper, and tie the paper on with string or put an elastic band around it.

6. Place the bowls in a steamer or set them into a pot of water. Steam them for 1 3/4 hours. Keep checking to make sure there's enough water in the pot.

7. When you remove them from the steam, let them cool before turning them out onto a plate.

1 1/4 cups (300 mL) whole wheat pastry flour

2 tsp (10 mL) baking powder

1/2 tsp (2 mL) nutmeg

1/2 tsp (2 mL) allspice

1/2 tsp (2 mL) cinnamon

1/2 tsp (2 mL) ginger powder

1 cup (240 mL) grated apple

1 cup (240 mL) grated carrot

1 cup (240 mL) grated potato

1/4–1/2 cup (60–120 mL) turbinado sugar

1 cup (240 mL) butter or ghee (page 41)

1 cup (240 mL) fine, dry bread crumbs

1 cup (240 mL) raisins

1 cup (240 mL) currants

1 cup (240 mL) finely chopped pitted dates

1/2 cup (120 mL) chopped walnuts

filo flowers

MAKES 1 DOZEN

These are so beautiful! This is Vasudev's invention ... not difficult, but the dessert is so yummy that Vasudev, a popular cook at the Centre, has to turn down proposals of marriage each time he makes them for our guests.

1. In a saucepan, mix all the ingredients except, obviously, the filo and ghee or melted butter. Cover and simmer for 40 to 50 minutes until the mixture is reduced.

Making flowers:
1. Grease two 6-cup muffin tins.
2. Lay one sheet of filo pastry on a cutting board or counter and brush it with melted butter or ghee.
3. Repeat this 2 more times so that you have 3 sheets of buttered filo, one on top of the other.

4 cups (960 mL) cored and chopped pears (3 medium pears)
1 cup (240 mL) raspberries, fresh or frozen 1/2 tin (6 3/4 oz) (200 mL) coconut milk or 1 cup (240 mL) rice milk and 4 Tbsp (60 mL) maple syrup
2 tsp (10 mL) cinnamon
1/4 tsp (1 mL) cardamom
1/4 tsp (1 mL) nutmeg
Pinch cloves

10 sheets filo pastry
1/4- 1/3 cup melted butter or ghee (page 41)

TIPS   SERVING

• Serve with whipped cream and a drizzle of Chocolate Sauce (page 128) to make a sinfully rich dessert.

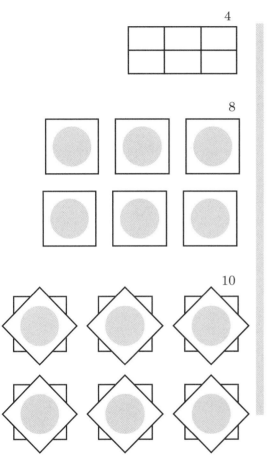

4. Cut the filo layers into 6 rectangles.

5. Repeat for the second muffin tin.

6. Place each small rectangle (of all 3 layers) into the bottom of a muffin cup, and press it into the cup.

7. Bake these at 375°F (190°C) for 3 to 4 minutes, until they're lightly browned.

8. Remove the muffin tins from the oven and fill the cups about two-thirds full with the filling, using 1/4 to 1/3 cup (60–80 mL) of filling for each cup.

9. Prepare two more sheets of filo, buttering them and laying one on top of the other. Cut these into six rectangles, just like the other ones.

10. Place each rectangle diagonally over the ones in the muffin tins to create a flower effect, pressing the middle down over the filling.

11. Repeat for the second muffin tin.

12. Bake these at 375°F (190°C) for 5 to 7 minutes, until the filo flowers are browned.

13. Remove them from the muffin tins and serve them topped with whipped cream and fresh fruit or whipped cream and Chocolate Sauce (page 128).

creamy chocolate pudding

SERVES 8-10

Absolutely delicious! You must use the best Belgian chocolate to ensure complete success.

4 1/2 cups (1.08 L) silken tofu
(3 boxes)

2/3 cup (160 mL) Belgian chocolate
chunks

1 tsp (5 mL) vanilla extract

1. Melt the chocolate in a double boiler.
2. Blend the melted chocolate, tofu, and vanilla in a food processor.
3. Serve at room temperature or chilled.

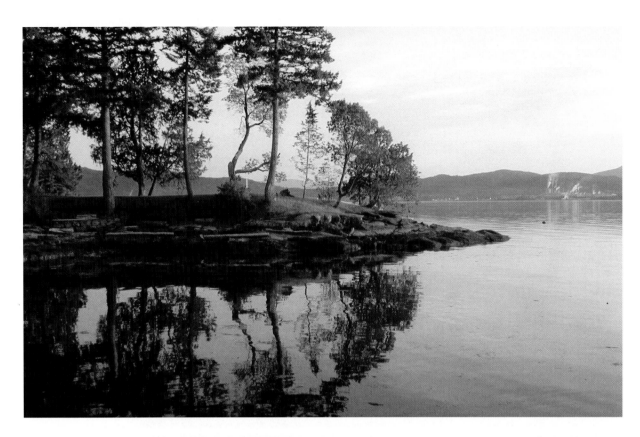

Quiet waters at
Sunset Point.

A contemplative
moment on the
Centre grounds.

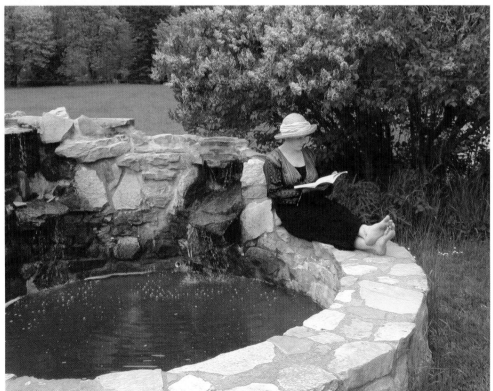

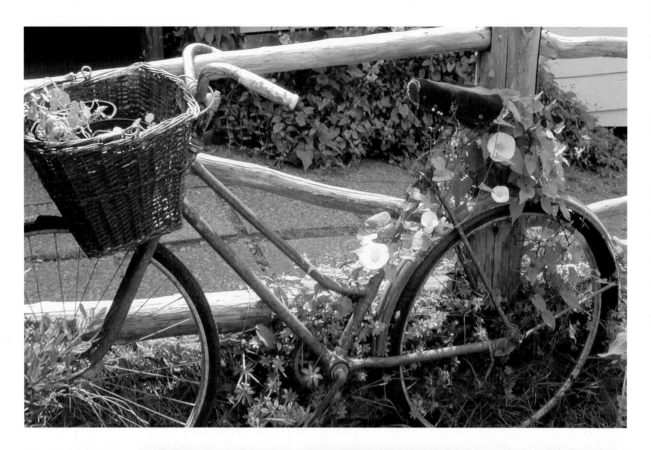

An old bike that is more lawn ornament than transportation these days.

Deer are a common sight in the meadows around the Centre.

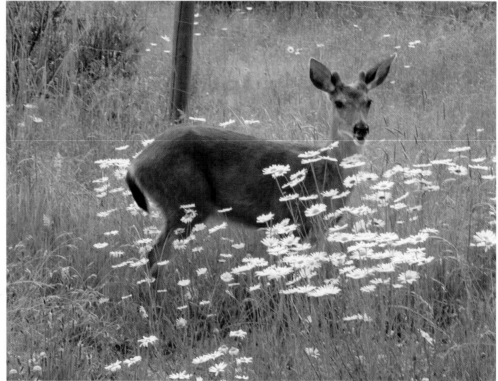

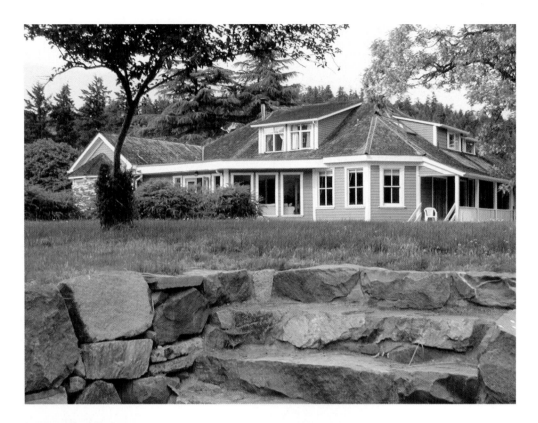

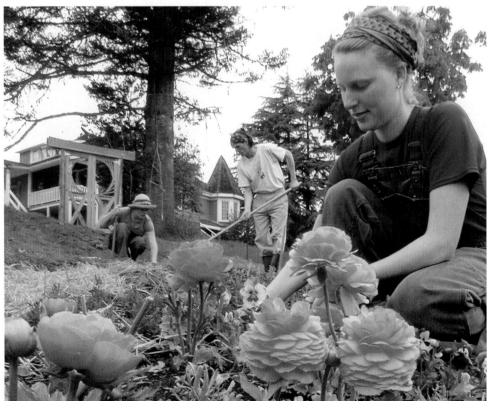

The Salt Spring Centre.

Everyone helps out in the garden.

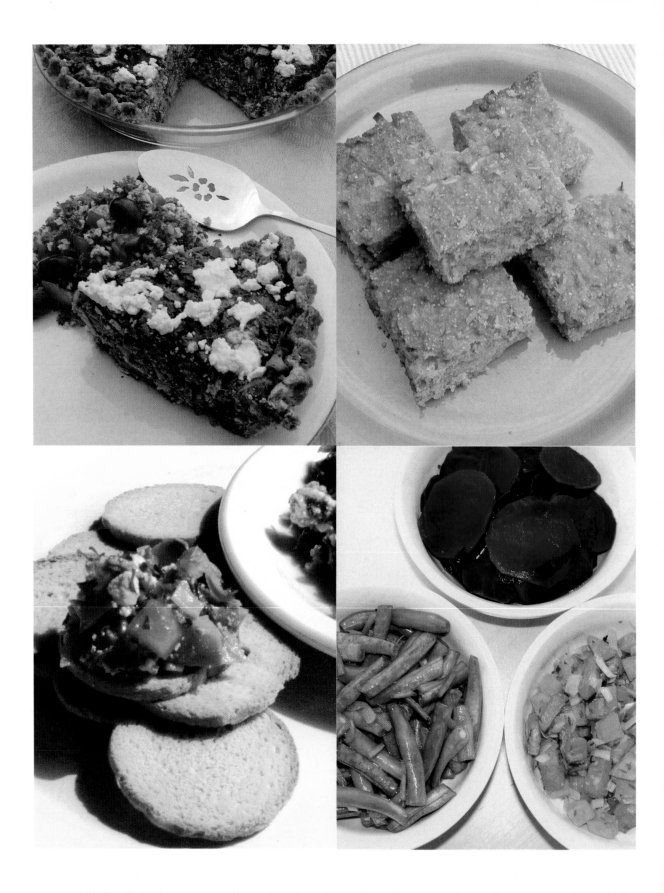

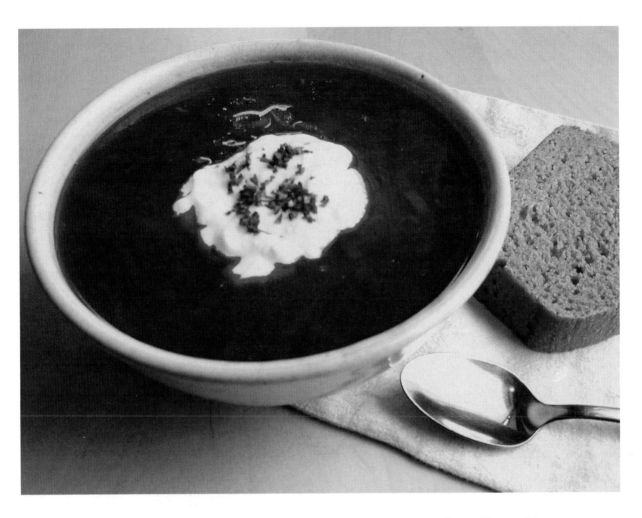

(above) A beautiful colour, Borscht is a hearty and delicious soup. Served here with yogurt and herbs (p. 14). (opposite page, clockwise from top left) Nayana's Mediterranean Tofu Quiche (p. 28) with Lebanese Tabouli (p. 66); Ann's Jalapeno Cornbread (p. 94); Three vegetables: The Beet Goes On (p. 52), Mary's Ginger Yams (p. 57), Zesty Ginger Beans (p. 56); Mushroom-Feta Topping (p. 93)

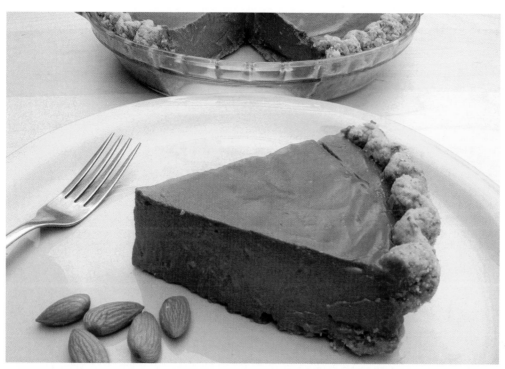

Velvet Chocolate Pie (p. 123)

Very Berry Frappé (p. 126) with Poppy Seed Cookies (p. 119)

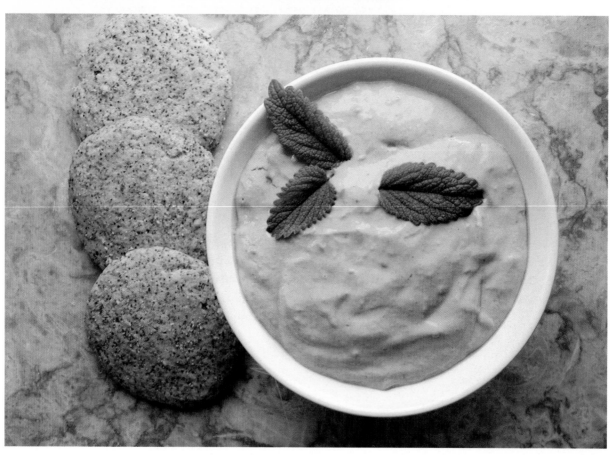

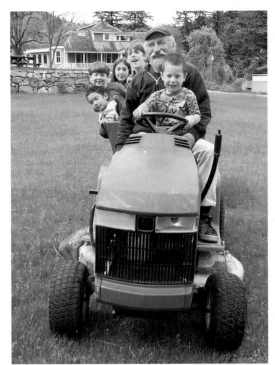

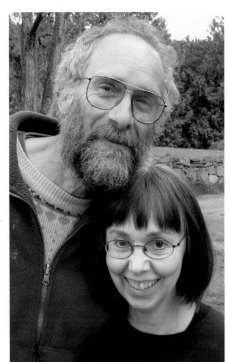

The kids love to take a ride.

Smiling faces from the Centre family.

Tomato plants in the greenhouse.

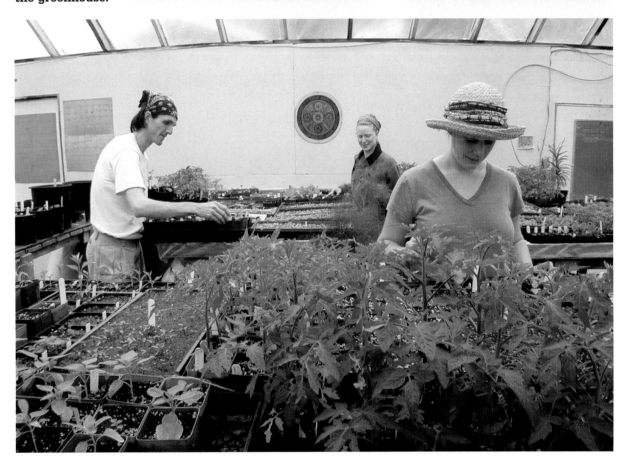

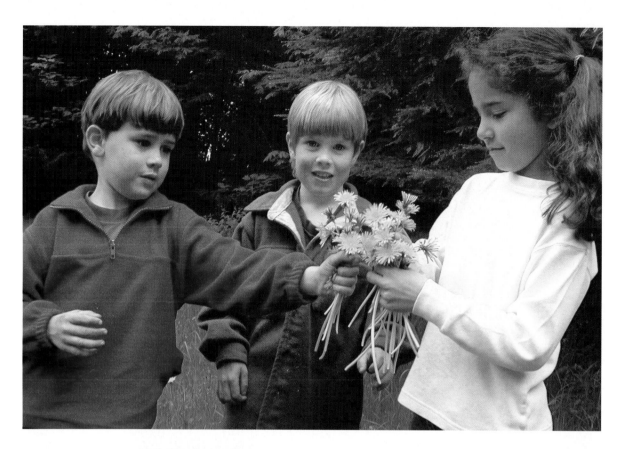

Children from the Centre school on the Woodland Trail.

Satellite Channel, with Mount Baker in the distance.

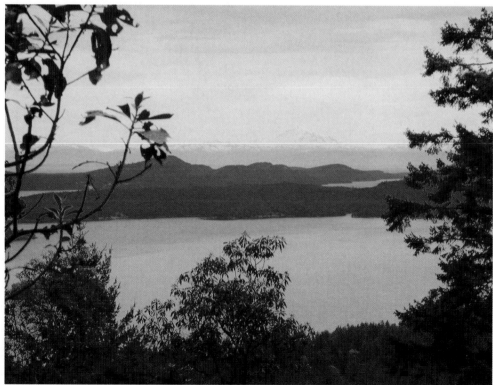

poppy seed cookies

MAKES 2 DOZEN

Mohn cookies for those in the know. For the rest of us, these are traditional Jewish poppy seed cookies.

1. Cream the butter and sugar, then add the vanilla and milk or soymilk.
2. Mix the flour, baking powder, salt, and poppy seeds. Mix this with the butter-sugar mixture.
3. Mix together the dry and wet ingredients.
4. Chill the dough for about half an hour, until it's firm enough to handle.
5. Roll the dough into small balls and press them onto an oiled cookie sheet.
6. Bake at 350°F (180°C) for 25 to 30 minutes.

1 cup (240 mL) butter

3/4 cup (180 mL) turbinado sugar

2 tsp (10 mL) vanilla extract

1/4 cup (60 mL) milk or soymilk

2 cups (480 mL) whole wheat pastry flour

2 tsp (10 mL) baking powder

Pinch salt

1/2 cup (120 mL) poppy seeds

THE DAY SHARADA MADE THESE, her friend Barry showed up, and she offered him a cookie. "Mohn cookies!" he exclaimed. I haven't had mohn cookies in years!" After tasting one, he proclaimed them better than his grandmother's. (Apologies to Barry's grandmother.)

TIPS
WHEAT-FREE

• To make these cookies wheat-free, replace the wheat flour with brown rice flour.

• Also, soak 4 tablespoons (60 mL) ground flaxseeds in 1/4 cup (60 mL) hot water for 15 minutes, and add to the wet ingredients.

rajani's baklava

Rajani is another of our multi-talented Centre family, being a health therapist and a cook. This is her double-jeopardy baklava—so sweetly delicious you might find yourself swinging from the chandeliers.

1. Melt 6 tablespoons (90 mL) butter or ghee in a saucepan.
2. Add the sugar, water, ground almonds, and lemon juice.
3. Cook this mixture slowly over medium-low heat until the sugar has fully dissolved, stirring frequently.
4. Add the cinnamon and cardamom, and mix it in.
5. Oil a 9 x 12 inch (23 x 30 cm) cake pan.
6. Lay one sheet of filo pastry on a cutting board or counter. Brush it with melted butter or ghee. Do the same with 5 more sheets of filo, placing one on top of the other to make a stack of 6 sheets of filo, each one brushed with butter or ghee.
7. Place the 6 layers of filo in the bottom of the baking pan, and spread half the almond mixture evenly over the filo.
8. Repeat this process with 6 more sheets of filo and the rest of the almond mixture.
9. Then add one more layer of 6 sheets of buttered filo on the top. If the filo is bigger than the pan, fold the ends back so it fits in the pan. Then brush the top of the filo with yet more melted butter or ghee.
10. Bake at 375°F (190°C) for 25 minutes or until the filo begins to turn golden brown.
11. When the baklava is done, remove it from the oven and score it in diamond shapes. Allow it to cool.

Filling:

6 Tbsp (90 mL) butter or ghee (page 41)

1 cup (240 mL) turbinado sugar

1 cup (240 mL) hot water

3 cups (720 mL) ground almonds

3 Tbsp (45 mL) lemon juice

1 Tbsp (15 mL) cinnamon

2 Tbsp (30 mL) cardamom

18 sheets filo pastry

1/3–1/2 cup (80–120 mL) melted butter or ghee (page 41)

Syrup for the top of the baklava:

1/2 cup (120 mL) turbinado sugar

1/2 cup (120 mL) water

Juice of 1 lemon

1/2 cup (120 mL) liquid honey

Syrup:

1. In a saucepan, cook the sugar, water, and lemon juice over medium-low heat for about 5 minutes.

2. Pour it into a bowl and let it cool. Then add the liquid honey and stir well.

3. Pour the syrup over the pan of baklava and spread it evenly. Let it stand at least 4 hours before serving—overnight is even better.

seven dwarf pudding

Very rich—a little will go a long way. But why is it called Seven Dwarf Pudding? Read the story below.

1/2 cup (120 mL) pitted dates

1 cup (240 mL) pitted prunes

1/2 cup (120 mL) water

3 Tbsp (45 mL) fresh lemon juice

1 medium banana

Grated rind of one orange

Juice of one lemon

2 cups (480 mL) whipping cream

1. In a saucepan, cook the dates, prunes, water, and 3 tablespoons (45 mL) lemon juice until the dates and prunes are soft.

2. In a food processor, blend the date-prune mixture with the banana, grated orange rind, and the juice of one lemon. Then pour it into a mixing bowl.

3. Whip the cream separately, and gently fold it into the date-prune mixture. If there seems to be too much whipping cream for your taste (it is very rich), don't mix it all in. Keep some to serve on top to those who aren't worried about calories.

YEARS AGO, WHEN NAYANA (of Mediterranean Tofu Quiche fame) was a little girl, she was helping Rajani prepare dinner for the community. Nayana's dad, Sid, kept coming into the kitchen with quizzes for Nayana, one of which was to name the seven dwarfs. Having Sid for a dad enabled her to name all seven dwarfs quickly while Rajani puzzled over them. When they had finished preparing the main part of the meal, they turned their attention to dessert. What else but Seven Dwarf Pudding! And now ... can you name the seven dwarfs?

Answer: The seven dwarfs are Doc, Happy, Sleepy, Sneezy, Bashful, Grumpy, and Dopey.

velvet chocolate pie

Tofu plus cream cheese combine to make a stunningly delicious chocolate pie, especially if you use the Almond Pie Crust (page 104).

1. In a saucepan, dissolve the sugar in the milk or rice milk over medium-low heat, and then allow it to cool.

2. Blend all the ingredients in a food processor until smooth.

3. Pour the mixture into a prepared Almond Pie Crust (page 104) that's been pre-baked at 350°F (180°C) for 10 to 12 minutes.

4. Turn the heat down to 325°F (165°C) and put the pie in the oven to bake for 30 minutes or until the crust is golden brown.

1 1/4 cups (300 mL) turbinado sugar
3/4 cup (180 mL) milk, rice milk, or soymilk
3 cups (720 mL) silken tofu
  (2 boxes)
3/4 cup (180 mL) cocoa powder
1 cup (240 mL) cream cheese
2 Tbsp (30 mL) arrowroot powder

trifle

Pretty and delicious—with many variations. If you're not a big coconut fan, use milk, rice milk, or soymilk to make the custard, and add 3 teaspoons (15 mL) of vanilla. Try using sugar instead of maple syrup, and use any cake or fruit.

1. Pour 1/2 cup (120 mL) of pineapple juice into the bottom of a large bowl.
2. Slice the cake into 1/4 inch (0.5 cm) slices and place a layer of cake on the bottom of the bowl over the juice. Spread 1/4 cup (60 mL) of jam or preserves over the cake.
3. Then make layers of fruit using half the peaches, pineapple, and banana, spreading the pieces over the jam/preserves.

1/2 cup (120 mL) pineapple juice
1/4–1/2 of an 8 x 8 inch white
  or angel food cake (see sidebar)
1/2 cup (120 mL) jam or preserves
1 cup (240 mL) thinly sliced fresh
  peaches or 19-oz tin (540 mL)
  thinly sliced canned peaches
19-oz tin (540 mL) pineapple bits
1 mango, peeled, thinly sliced
3 bananas, thinly sliced
1/2 cup (120 mL) custard powder
1/4 cup (60 mL) maple syrup
2 13.5-oz tins (800 mL) coconut milk
1 1/2 cups (360 mL) rice milk
1/4 cup (60 mL) toasted almonds or
  coconut

TIPS   VARIATIONS

• White cake or angel food cake is traditional, but feel free to try others. We've made delicious trifle with chocolate cake.
• To make the trifle wheat-free, use a wheat-free cake, cookies, or wafers.

4. Repeat cake, jam, and fruit layers.

5. In a saucepan, mix the custard powder with 1/3 cup coconut milk (or rice milk), stirring until smooth. (If using sugar or vanilla, mix them in also). Add the rest of the coconut milk and rice milk. Cook over medium-low heat, stirring constantly, until the mixture thickens and begins to boil, then remove from heat.

6. Pour the custard over the layers in the bowl, poking holes with a knife to make sure the custard goes through all the layers.

7. Sprinkle the toasted crushed almonds or toasted coconut over the top.

8. Refrigerate overnight.

A TRUE STORY FROM JULIE, SHARADA'S MOM. When she was first married, many years ago, Julie knew that in her new husband's family, trifle was the traditional birthday dessert—but she'd never tasted trifle, much less made one.

A week before Irv's birthday in that first year of their marriage, a package arrived in the mail for her. In the box was Irv's mom's trifle recipe along with all the necessary ingredients, already measured out. Julie says that the look on Irv's face when she brought out the big bowl of trifle was priceless. Although they're both in their eighties now, the tradition continues.

very berry frappé

Masquerades as a sherbet.

3 cups (720 mL) frozen berries
(raspberries, blueberries, or
strawberries)
3 cups (720 mL) silken tofu
(2 boxes)
1/4 cup (60 mL) soy or rice milk
1/2–3/4 cup (120–180 mL) maple
syrup

1. Blend all the ingredients in a food processor until smooth.
2. Taste for sweetness. Raspberries will need more sweetener than blueberries or strawberries.
3. Serve at room temperature or chill in glass bowls before serving. Beautiful garnished with a mint leaf.

winter squash pie

Don't be deceived by the humble-sounding name. This pie is even more delicious than its relative, pumpkin pie. (Pumpkin is a squash, too!)

1. To cook the squash, cut it in half, remove the seeds, and turn it upside down in a baking pan with a bit of water. Bake it at 400°F (205°C) for about half an hour or until it's soft.

2. In a saucepan, simmer the milk (or rice milk or soymilk) and sugar until the sugar dissolves.

3. When the squash is done, scoop the pulp out and blend it with all the other ingredients in a food processor until it's smooth.

4. Line a pie plate with Almond Pie Crust (page 104), and pre-bake the crust at 350°F (180°C) for 12 minutes.

5. Remove the pie plate from the oven, and pour the filling into the pre-baked pie shell.

6. Reduce the heat to 325°F (165°C) and bake the pie for 40 minutes.

1 large winter squash (Hubbard or butternut) (about 3 1/2 cups [840 mL] puréed)

1 cup (240 mL) milk, rice milk, or soymilk

3/4 cup (180 mL) turbinado sugar

1 1/2 cups (360 mL) silken tofu (1 box)

1 Tbsp (15 mL) cinnamon

1 tsp (5 mL) cloves

1 1/2 tsp (7 mL) powdered ginger

1/4 tsp (1 mL) salt

3 tsp (15 mL) vanilla extract

mary's chocolate sauce

Great on cakes, ice cream, and Filo Flowers (page 116). Can be made as a sauce or an icing.

1 cup (240 mL) butter or
  ghee (page 41)
2/3 cup (160 mL) turbinado sugar
3 Tbsp (45 mL) cocoa powder
1/3 cup (80 mL) milk, rice milk,
  or soymilk
2 tsp (10 mL) vanilla extract

1. Melt the butter or ghee in a saucepan. Then add the sugar and cocoa and mix in with a whisk.
2. Over medium-low heat, bring it to a boil and cook it for 2 to 3 minutes, stirring frequently.
3. Whisk in the milk and vanilla. Leaving the heat set to medium-low, bring the mixture to a full boil again, and cook for 5 to 10 minutes (until the sugar dissolves). It will thicken a bit, more if you cook it longer. To make it thick enough to use as an icing, make sure you cook it for the full 10 minutes.
4. Pour warm (if using as a sauce) or chill (if using as icing).

lemon sauce I

MAKES 2 1/2 CUPS (600 ML)

The dairy version—soymilk won't work. If you'd prefer to avoid the cream, go immediately to Lemon Sauce II, opposite.

1. In a saucepan, mix the cream and arrowroot while the cream is cold.

2. Add the remaining ingredients and simmer over low heat until the sauce thickens, stirring constantly.

2 cups (480 mL) light cream

2 Tbsp (30 mL) arrowroot powder

1/2 cup (120 mL) fresh lemon juice
(3 lemons)

1/2 cup (120 mL) turbinado sugar

1/4 cup (60 mL) water

lemon sauce II

The cream-free version, just as tasty as Lemon Sauce I. Definitely not second best. This is the sauce that's traditionally served over Mayana's Gran's Carrot Pudding (page 115).

3 cups (720 mL) water

3/4 cup (180 mL) turbinado sugar

3 Tbsp (45 mL) arrowroot powder dissolved in 1 Tbsp (15 mL) cold water

3 Tbsp (45 mL) butter or ghee (page 41)

3 Tbsp (45 mL) fresh lemon juice

2–3 Tbsp (30–45 mL) grated lemon rind

1 Tbsp (15 mL) vanilla extract

1. Boil the water in a saucepan, turn the heat to low, add the sugar, and stir to dissolve it.

2. Mix the arrowroot and cold water in a bowl. Remove some of the sugar-water mixture and mix it with the arrowroot mixture. Once it's mixed, pour it back into the saucepan, and stir until it's thickened.

3. Remove the saucepan from the heat, and add the remaining ingredients.

raspberry-blueberry sauce

Lovely colour, sweetly delicious. Not only does it complement the Cheesecake on page 111, but it also goes well with yogurt, ice cream, or porridge.

1. In a saucepan, simmer the berries, water, and maple syrup or sugar for about 10 minutes until the berries are reduced.

2. In a bowl, mix the arrowroot and the cold water, then add it and the vanilla to the berries.

3. Simmer another 10 to 15 minutes until the mixture thickens.

4. If you're using this as a cheesecake topping, let it cool a bit before spreading it on the cheesecake, but not too long or it will be too thick to spread.

1 cup (240 mL) raspberries

2 cups (480 mL) blueberries

1/2 cup (120 mL) water

1/4–1/3 cup (60–80 mL) maple syrup
   or turbinado sugar

3 1/4 Tbsp (48 mL) arrowroot

1/2 cup (120 mL) cold water

1 Tbsp (15 mL) vanilla extract

TIPS   VARIATIONS

• You can use all raspberries or all blueberries—or any other berries.

• Raspberries generally require more sweetener than the others.

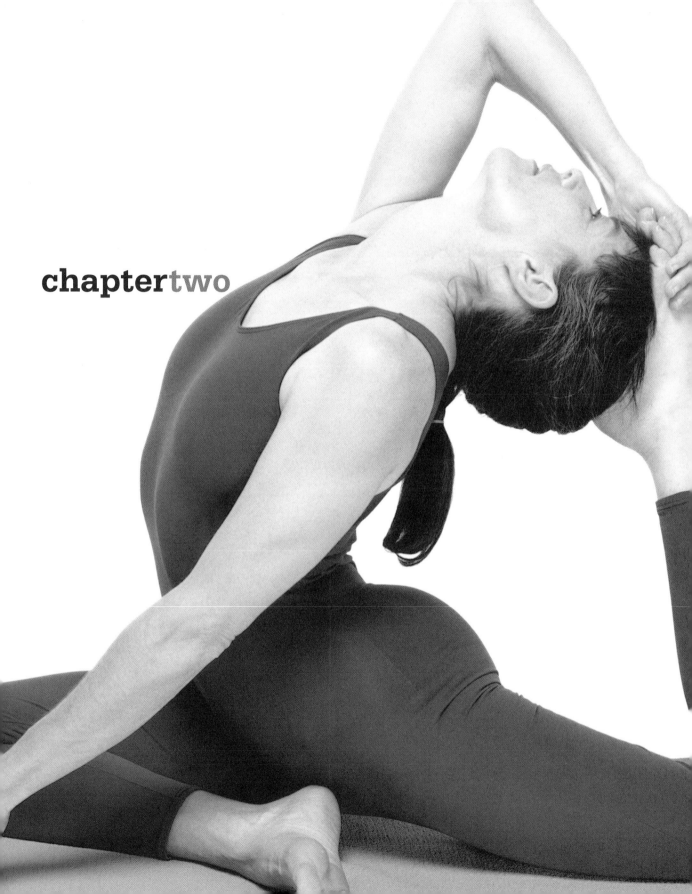

chaptertwo

yoga philosopy and practice:
more than standing on your head

What Is Yoga?

WHEN YOU HEAR THE WORD YOGA, WHAT DO YOU THINK OF? If you live anywhere in the Western world, chances are you think of exercises. It's not surprising. Many neighbourhoods offer yoga classes in the local community centre or YMCA. Yoga, however, is more than standing on your head or twisting your body into a pretzel shape.

Perhaps you go to a yoga class once a week, and you really like your teacher. You enjoy the stretching and the relaxation. Your yoga teacher begins the class with a short meditation and ends the class by chanting *Om*. It's quite pleasant, but you wonder what it's about. Does it mean you're getting into some New Age cultish thing? Is it okay to be doing this? You're not particularly religious, but it feels a bit odd to be doing this Eastern practice. You're not alone. Here's what one yoga student had to say:

> When I first went to a gathering at which people were singing ancient Sanskrit chants, I felt vaguely uncomfortable. I felt somehow that I was betraying my own heritage, though I don't think I really understood that at the time. All I knew was that all this chanting was not something my parents or anyone else in my family would feel comfortable with.

Yoga is not the same as Hinduism, although yoga often appears clothed in Hindu trappings because of its origins in India. Yoga is not a religion and does not contradict any belief system, so whether you're Christian, Jewish, or any other faith, or whether you consider yourself an agnostic or an atheist, it doesn't matter. Yoga practice can be done by anyone; its purpose is to help us find peace, and peace is the same for everyone.

The yoga postures, or asanas, which may be familiar to many people, are part of a larger system that originated in India thousands of years ago. The postures were first developed to condition the body, enabling it to sit in a meditation posture for the purpose of stilling the mind and finding peace.

Searching for Meaning

Regardless of their culture, people search for meaning in their lives. Many systems have been developed to explain why we are here, what life is about, and what we can do to live happier lives. Yoga philosophy and psychology address the questions that people have wrestled with in every age.

Everybody wants to be happy. We try hard. We latch onto things and people that please us and avoid those that don't. If we manage to feel okay more than we feel miserable, we say we're happy—but we have those moments when we sense there should be more to life. It hits a lot of people in midlife, though it can happen at any age. There's a sense that we've been living our lives with some essential ingredient missing. Although we may have material comforts, a decent job, a family we get along with most of the time, and friends to spend time with, there's a feeling that we're not fully alive.

Although uncomfortable, this is not necessarily a bad thing. It all depends on what we do with these anxious feelings. Ignoring them is one option, although it doesn't work very well since the feelings tend to seep out somewhere. Trying to understand what's happening under the surface of our lives is more productive and definitely more interesting.

Let's look at the way we live our lives. There are many variations of course, but most of us want to accomplish something in our work, have loving and supportive relationships, good health, and physical comfort. There's nothing wrong with these goals, and in this part of the world we have the freedom to pursue them. Yet for all our freedom, we sense that we're living unfulfilled lives. Why? What limits us? It's easy to look outside ourselves for something or someone to blame for our discontent. In fact, most of us are experts at laying blame elsewhere.

Sometimes we look into the workings of our own hearts and minds through some sort of counselling or therapy. This course of action can be enormously beneficial, and can help us get perspective on the difficulties in our lives and deal with the challenges we face.

The yogic way of dealing with our dissatisfactions is to seek to understand the workings of our own minds. Debates about nature or nurture aside, the fact is that we act the way we've been conditioned to act. It's as if we've been given our roles (via our parents, our genes, our natural tendencies), and we play them well. We have varying abilities, talents, opportunities, and scenarios, none of which we have any control over, and we let ourselves be defined by them. When we encounter some difficulty in life, we deal with it the way we've always dealt with it, the way we've learned to deal with it. In fact, we do everything that way.

If we watch our thoughts for a period of time, we'll begin to realize that we think the same thoughts over and over. There are variations to be sure, but we tend to recycle the same material again and again. The people around us come to expect us to behave in a particular way, as we do of them. How could we do otherwise? We can certainly gain new skills and become more sophisticated in our communications, but the thoughts are still the same, though perhaps cloaked in cleverer dialogue.

The "I–Me–Mine" Syndrome

Whatever our role in life, we are all ruled by one main thought–theme: "Is this good for me? Is this going to make me look good? Is this going to make me happy?" If we pay attention, we'll notice that everything we do, every thought we think, is about "me." I, me, mine, just like the old Beatles tune. Does this thing make me happy? Does this person make me happy?

It's natural to want what makes us happy, or at least what we think will make us happy. It could be anything—a new car, house, toy, relationship (you name it, somebody wants it). The problem is that what each of us wants may conflict with what someone else wants. We're not all going to get what we want. And of course, when we don't get what we want, we have fairly predictable patterns of behaviour to show how we feel about it.

Although we understand intellectually that other people have needs, we usually operate as if we're the centre of the universe. Lovely as the dream of living in peace and harmony is, it can't happen if each of us is living a life of "What's in it for me?" If that's the pattern all of us operate by, how can we ever find real peace and happiness?

The good news is that happiness is possible. We can live our lives peacefully and happily, with a feeling of fulfillment. As with anything else that's worth doing, changing our patterns of behaviour takes commitment and practice. It's not an instant fix. Anyone who's ever studied a new skill understands that to get better at something, you need to practise. Nobody starts out playing Mozart or Bach masterfully. You start where you are. "Where we are" may be confused, anxious, sad, restless, or sick. That's okay. You start where you are. This is not about judgment. We already have enough ways to make ourselves feel bad. Anything that we do toward creating peace is useful.

We all face difficulties in life; no one is exempt. To be human is to deal with challenges, some simple, some difficult (and some very difficult), but we seem to need them in order to grow. During the process of putting this book together, many people shared stories of their struggles, which we are happy to share with you.

It had been a terrible year, and I wasn't coping very well. During this time I had a private interview with my spiritual teacher, who told me that my anger was the cause of my family's problems. Once I stopped crying and shaking, I asked him what I could do. He told me to pretend to be a separate person from the person who is angry. That angry person is over there and you are here. I tried it and the anger simply seemed to melt. I can't always do it, but I'm getting better at it.

Why Practise Yoga?

People practise yoga for many different reasons. People often begin yoga classes because they've heard yoga postures will help them become fit—just like going to the gym, but with more stretching. And it works. Doing yoga postures regularly can enhance health on many levels—stretching muscles, increasing circulation, enhancing energy. That in itself is a good thing, but it's useful to understand that the main purpose of asanas, or postures, is to prepare the mind and body for meditation. Other practices, such as pranayama (breathing practices), also help calm the mind as preparation for meditation.

The word *meditation* is tossed around lightly these days, and is used to describe some practices that are more properly described as "relaxation." Now relaxation is a good thing, and most of us could use more of it, but we also need to know that that's not what meditation is.

According to the Yoga Sutras of Patanjali, ancient texts from India that expound the philosophy and practice of yoga, "Yoga is the control of thought waves in the mind." What exactly does that mean? It means we practise various methods of breath control and concentration to still the mind so that our thoughts are not running wild as they usually do. This is a tall order.

In the beginning, we may spend a great deal of time just sitting, looking as though we're meditating, while our thoughts are completely out of control. In fact, they're no more out of control than they usually are; they follow their usual habit of jumping from one fantasy to another. But in the busyness of our day–to–day lives, we don't notice how wayward our thoughts really are. After all, it's normal.

After regularly sitting for meditation practice, however, we catch glimpses of these unruly minds of ours. We may also have many moments of "spacing out"—suddenly finding ourselves compiling grocery lists or planning what we're going to wear to the party next week or fantasizing about what we're going to tell the boss when we get to work.

Just like puppies that run after anything that moves, our minds will follow any thought. Just like puppies, our minds need to be trained. Unfortunately they tend to be more resistant to training than puppies are.

So what's wrong with having wild puppy minds? Minds jumping all over the place can't lead to contentment and peace. Yoga philosophy, as expounded in the Yoga Sutras, teaches about the nature of the mind and then proceeds to tell us what we can do about the predicament of having endlessly chattering minds.

Yoga's Ethical Underpinnings

Yoga is a philosophy that is intended to be lived by real people. As such, yoga encompasses principles by which people can live, or strive to live. These principles include yamas (restraints) and niyamas (observances).

The Restraints (Yamas)
1. non-harming (ahimsa)
2. truthfulness (satya)
3. non-stealing (asteya)
4. sexual continence (brahmacharya)
5. non-hoarding (aparigraha)

The Observances (Niyamas)
1. cleanliness and purity (shaucha)
2. contentment (santosha)
3. austerity (tapas)
4. scriptural study and self-study (svadhyaya)
5. surrender to God (Ishvarapranidhana)

The very first restraint, and the foundation for all the others, is non-harming. This does not simply mean not hitting each other or yelling at each other. It goes far beyond that. We are to endeavour to live without harmful actions, words, and even thoughts. That means not even thinking negative thoughts about others—or even ourselves. This, by

itself, is a lifetime practice. Just think—if we could truly live without harming others (and that's not just human lives, but all of this planet and beyond), what would be left? Without enmity, what's left is love.

> *In learning to practise non-violence, I can see that it begins in my mind, with my thoughts. If I cannot attain peace in my thoughts, then I cannot attain it in my life. And so, posted on my mirrors, fridge, TV, and altar are the words "Practise non-violent thoughts." This does not mean don't kick the postman. It means don't kick myself for not doing this or that, or for doing this or that wrong. It is only when I learn to treat myself gently and with love that I'm able to treat others this way and create non-violence, love, and gentleness in my outer world.*

The second restraint is truthfulness, which means cultivating honesty on all levels. We are to avoid deceiving others. At first glance, this seems simple—but what about the tendency to exaggerate or slant a story to make us look good? Truthfulness also includes not deceiving ourselves; this is even more challenging.

Non-stealing, of course, includes not taking things that belong to someone else, but it also includes not taking other people's ideas or accepting credit for something that we really don't deserve credit for.

The concept of sexual continence is probably the most misunderstood of the restraints. It is not intended that we all live like monks and nuns, but rather that we control our impulses and limit our desires in order to redirect our minds. In this part of the world, that is an odd concept. There's not much in our culture that supports the limiting of desires, but even the choice to be with one partner is a limitation. Above all, limiting or reducing desires is about cultivating an attitude of peace and contentment.

Non-hoarding, though easier to understand, also goes against the grain of our culture, which is, after all, built on satisfying our desires, getting more, more, more. Placing limits on our desires allows us to choose more consciously.

For one who wants to limit the distractions in the mind, these restraints provide the foundation.

The observances begin with cleanliness, which refers to cleanliness of the body and purity of mind. Cleanliness of the body is fairly straightforward, but what does purity of mind mean? It means cultivating positive qualities, practising responding with kindness and compassion.

And contentment—who even knew you could practise it? Most of us assume that contentment is the end result rather than something we can actually cultivate. But if we choose a course of action and do the best we can, what more can we do? Contentment means accepting what life is, and that is something we can practise.

Then there's austerity, that limiting-desires thing again, hardly popular these days. It doesn't mean wearing hair shirts or sleeping on a bed of nails; rather, it's about living a disciplined life, not indulging in whatever whims appear in the mind.

Scriptural study is more than book study. It includes self-study, watching the habits of our minds and reflecting on who we are. What is "watching the mind" and how can we do it? Although we do so much without awareness of our motives, we can begin to notice what's going on behind the scenes. We live our lives as the protagonist in our own drama, but we can learn to step off the stage at times and be in the audience. It can be very revealing (though it may make the protagonist appear somewhat less attractive).

The concept of surrender to God is difficult for many people to understand. Our culture has mixed feelings about God. While many adhere to traditional ideas about God, many do not; many question the very existence of God. Your own nature and background determine your beliefs.

Regardless of religious beliefs, anyone can practise surrender to God.

According to yoga teachings, what we're surrendering is our self-importance. We recognize that we are limited by our self-concepts, and are guided most often by our self-interest. In surrendering to God, we channel our energies toward the realization of truth, universal Self, or God, allowing ourselves to be guided by that rather than by our individual egos.

Surrender to God can be understood to mean acceptance of that over which we have no control. Things happen. The universe is neither benevolent nor malevolent. Life is just what it is. If we can accept that and stop struggling so hard, we can be content. This doesn't mean that we don't continue to do what we need to do; it means rather that we do all we can do and accept that the results are not up to us.

I have a chronic illness that is turning out to be an advanced course in "surrender to God" practice. On the days when my body is racked with symptoms—pain, shaking, cramping, etc.—I try to be totally in the moment, experiencing each moment as it passes, praying for God's support and grace to help me make it through as best I can.

Different Natures, Different Paths

We have different natures and tendencies, and we don't all enjoy doing the same things. Whatever your temperament, you will be drawn to one of yoga's three main paths. If you're the studious type there's Jnana (pronounced *gyana*) Yoga, the path of intellectual inquiry. If you're filled with gratitude and love there's Bhakti Yoga, the yoga of devotion (see Forgiveness Asanas, page 172). If you'd prefer to be busy, actively "doing something" rather than immersed in study or prayer, there's Karma Yoga, the yoga of action.

The beauty of the system is that all the ways work. What does that mean, they "work"? What are they working at? They're working on the mind, gradually wearing away the prickly edges of our egos.

Karma Yoga, for example, doesn't just mean working; it means doing work as a duty. Duty is another one of those words that aren't very popular in this culture. It has a Victorian flavour to it. But what it really means is that you do what needs to be done, period. If the floor needs sweeping, you sweep it; if the dishes need washing, you wash them; if the baby's diaper needs changing, you change it. You don't do any of these things in a robot-like fashion. You do them with all the enthusiasm and good-heartedness that you can muster. And then that's it. You don't expect anyone to say what a great guy you are—"Wow! You changed the baby's diaper. Aren't you great!" You do what you do with diligence and joy (if you can) and then you move on to the next thing. The point is that you don't do it for a result—not for a paycheque, for praise, or for recognition.

Of course, most of us are not so evolved that we can do that all the time, but that's the intent, and sometimes it happens. The problem is that when we realize we've just done something selflessly, the voice of self-congratulation chimes in "Wow! Am I ever selfless." Oops. Back to square one, but don't worry, there are endless opportunities.

I have a habit of responding to requests by saying, "For you, dear, anything." I say it (some would say much too often) so that I can forget what I want and just do what I can to help others. If I can convince myself of this, then the "I" shrinks. I've been asked if I mean it when I say "For you, dear, anything." Most times I do . . . when I'm not too busy doing what I want.

Ego, Desire, and Attachment: The Big Three

Our minds are very clever. The ego, which in its purest form is simply the sense of "I," has a habit of claiming everything for itself. That's why it's so hard to act in a truly selfless fashion. You do something kind for someone and the ego immediately congratulates itself.

It's not just in acts of kindness that the ego rears its head; it's present in negative actions, too. You make a mistake and the ego shows up again, this time to berate you: "I'm such a jerk! I never do anything right.

No wonder no one likes me." The ego wallows in self-pity, loving every moment of it.

Wait a minute, we hear you saying. Why would the ego enjoy self-flagellation? The ego likes it because it feels important: "No one is as miserable as I am." What the ego enjoys is separateness. When we feel miserable, we don't feel connected to anyone; we feel isolated. When we feel joyous and loving, we feel less separate and lonely and the ego feels less important.

Yoga says clearly that desires and attachments are trouble; that they keep us stuck in the realm of suffering; that they are, in fact, the cause of suffering. Ego, desire, and attachment—the big three. The "I, Me, Mine" theme of our lives ensures that we always want something. The something we want could be anything—a new car, a new relationship, or a piece of chocolate cheesecake.

Of course, we don't always get what we want, and then what happens? We feel disappointed, sad, or perhaps angry. But sometimes we do get what we want, and what happens then? We get attached, we want to keep it, we hold on for dear life and worry that we won't be able to keep the thing that we think is bringing us happiness.

What if we didn't have that angst? What if whatever happened, we'd still be okay?

A few years ago I was on my way to a mountain village market day in Guatemala. The early morning bus for which I had been waiting approached at a high speed, already crowded with vendors. Even before the bus slid to a halt, the driver's young assistant scrambled out the rear door and climbed up to the overhead roof rack and began to catch the bundles thrown up to him by the

embarking passengers. Being mistrustful of this overhead laissez-faire baggage system, I clutched my new and rather full backpack to my chest. As I boarded, I was stopped by the driver. He motioned me curtly to leave my backpack on the floor beside him just inside the front door. I took a few hesitant steps to the back and stood, all the seats already taken.

At each stop more passengers pressed onto the bus, pushing me farther and farther to the rear, separating me from my precious belongings. I became more and more apprehensive as my bag periodically disappeared from view.

Finally, the bus became so jammed that I lost sight of it altogether. I thought wildly of pushing my way forward, but that seemed not only embarrassing, but impossible.

Then, there was a very distinct moment when I realized that there was nothing I could do, and that worrying was not going to help. I just let go and surrendered to the situation. I turned my head to gaze out the window. There was the exquisite sight of the terraced mountainsides and the sun rising in a bright blue sky over the perfectly shaped cones of ancient volcanoes.

Every Moment Counts

One of the problems with holding on, apart from the tension and anxiety it creates, is that the things we are so attached to are, by their very nature, impossible to grasp. Everything we have and everything we want will one day break, decay, disappear, or die. Everything and everyone on this earth has a limited lifespan. Everything. Some lifespans are short and some are long, but they all end. And the truth is that even though we act as though everything is for keeps, deep down we know it's not. We ourselves will die. We don't like to think about it and we frequently act in ways that deny the existence of death, but in truth, none of us knows if we'll be here next year or even tomorrow.

Accepting this basic truth of life allows us to be present to what is right now. Yes, we have to make practical plans; this is not an invitation to laziness and the avoidance of responsibility. Rather, it's a reminder to be present at this very moment. Many of us are only partly here because our minds are already a few steps ahead—or absorbed in some memory.

Often we live our lives with gaps between the events that we count as real. Leaving the house in the morning, driving to work, become in-between moments that we don't count as real life. As we drive, how many of us are really somewhere else? But there really are no in-between moments; life is one seamless whole in which every moment counts. Our job is to be aware every moment.

I was scheduled to go to Vancouver on Wednesday for surgery to remove a growth on my thigh. I had gone the previous week for another MRI of my leg and a CT scan of my chest, as the form of cancer I had can spread to the lungs.

At 8:30 on Monday morning, the phone rang. It was the doctor's receptionist saying I had to come in for an appointment that afternoon. I asked if they had the results of the CT scan, and she answered yes but that I'd have to come in to discuss it with the doctor.

I was barely dressed, my shoelaces were undone, and the pain in my leg was so intense I couldn't sit comfortably anywhere. It was a dark, rainy November morning, and my spirits were as dark as the day. I thought, "My God, the cancer has spread to my lungs and he can't operate. It's all over."

On the ferry, the ship's captain stopped the boat and announced that there was a pod of killer whales on the starboard side of the ship. I couldn't walk well but I thought it might be my last chance to see Orcas. The rain was coming down in buckets, but I got out of the car with my husband and went to see the whales.

There was a family of Orcas—male, female, aunt, and baby. My tears joined the rain streaking down my cheeks. The whales came directly toward us, jumping up and going under, until a few feet from us they went under the ship. They surfaced again and were joined by two more pods of Orcas. I couldn't stop crying. As my tears flowed, I felt connected, at one with the whales, and the pain in my heart eased.

When we went back to the car I began to sob. My husband asked if I was okay. I nodded. I knew that whatever happened, it would be okay.

When our minds become agitated over something that's happening, it can be helpful to ask ourselves, "If I were to die in this moment, is this what I want to have in my mind?" And in that moment, we can choose to change the angle of our minds.

Recently a friend of mine passed away, and it was a source of deep reflection. Now whenever some event disturbs my peace of mind, I ask myself if this would be of great significance if I were dying.

Changing the Angle of the Mind

"The mind becomes serene by the cultivation of feelings of love for the happy, compassion for the suffering, delight for the virtuous, and indifference for the non-virtuous." This is one of the many methods for attaining peace taught in the Yoga Sutras.

Is that what we generally do? More typically, when we see someone who's happy, especially if we're less than happy, we're annoyed by the person's joyfulness. The bah-humbug! attitude. Think about how you react when a group of people is happily, and perhaps noisily, having fun when you're down in the dumps. Wouldn't it be great to be able to be happy that they're happy?

And what about compassion for the suffering? Chances are we can act compassionately sometimes, but what about the homeless person on the street who asks you for change, or even your own child (or your partner) who's feeling miserable and who's whining about some perceived injustice? Are we compassionate then?

And delight for the virtuous? Often we're irritated by them, and perhaps cynical about their goodness. Indifference for the non-virtuous? Hardly. We're usually more than ready to blame and seek blood.

Wouldn't it be wonderful to be able to respond with love and compassion? It takes work because we have to change the angle of our minds, something we're not used to doing. But the great thing is that if we consciously choose to respond more lovingly and compassionately, it changes us. We can, little by little, retrain these intractable minds of ours, and in doing so feel more peace.

Do we want to feel more peaceful? A lot of us think we need passion and attachments; that without them there wouldn't be much left, and our lives would be dull.

I had always lived life vividly. I viewed the agony of deep feelings of loss or despair as part of feeling alive, a necessary counterpart to the ecstatic joy of wonder or achievement, or just the basic excitement of good fun. My first response to yoga's suggestion that I live a life of balanced calm, maintaining a steady peace of mind, unexcited by highs or lows, was "Not for me, thanks!" But slowly I discovered that both my body and my mind were deeply attracted to the calm that certain yoga practices induced.

Peace doesn't mean boredom or indifference. It means stopping the war against others and ourselves—the judgment, criticism, anger, irritation, jealousy. Rather than implying that we can't enjoy life, it means that we truly can, without interference from our opinions.

Simplifying Life

One of the ways to move toward peace is to simplify our lives. We're not talking about moving to a cabin in the woods and living without electricity, but rather about limiting our desires. We complicate our lives unnecessarily, with things to have and things to do. Of course, there are things we have that make our lives easier, and that's fine. We have *them*; they don't have us. And then there are the things we do to fill in all the empty spaces in our lives. Many of us are obsessed with doing something every moment. Even when we rest our bodies, our minds continue churning out thoughts, keeping us busy.

Simplifying life means choosing what's important, and doing it with full awareness; being present in this moment rather than looking back or jumping ahead. Limiting desires can lead us to contentment. We don't have to occupy our minds with endless choices if we've already limited our choices to what we've decided is important. It's easier to make commitments if we've consciously chosen them rather than being tossed around by the waves of experience.

> *For a long time I felt like my "spiritual life" and my "worldly life" were separate. I grew up in a spiritual community; growing up it was clear to me that the Centre was my spiritual home. But how could I take the peace and simplicity I find there into the rest of my life? I'm in school 14 hours a day. I don't meditate regularly, I don't go to spiritual gatherings, I don't have an altar or pictures of a guru up all over my house.*
>
> *So how do I practise? I practise acceptance. Although I have a great love for God, I don't think about God daily in the form of chant or prayer. I try to live a life of service. As I get older, I decide again and again to live a spiritual life. I choose to allow the spiritual laws I'm familiar with to be present with me day to day. Why do I do this? It simplifies my life.*

Training the Puppy

We have wild puppy minds that need training, but where do we start? Watching the mind is a good place to begin. We can begin to retrain our minds by keeping an eye on them so that they can't continue to misbe-

have to quite the same degree.

When you catch yourself falling into a familiar pattern—criticizing someone because he disagrees with you, getting angry because you didn't get what you want, feeling sorry for yourself—whatever the pattern, you can stop yourself. Just say no, I'm not going there this time. Stop the video, rewind, and change the ending. Not easy, of course. Your ego will do everything in its power to convince you that you have every reason to feel sad or angry.

Keep watching. When you follow the ego's advice, do you feel connected to others, loving, peaceful? Or do you feel isolated from others? That's a clue. Don't expect to be able to do this all the time, and don't give yourself a hard time if you fail. That's just another voice of the ego, stopping you from feeling happy and peaceful.

> *I'm in the middle of a difficult divorce, and I'm striving to seek the light and the positive in this situation. When I find myself enticed into the negative—revenge, hate, and fear—I stop (or try to!) and take myself, my essential self, to a safe place where I can be soft but not sleepy and alert with no strain. I take several breaths, and when I'm ready, I invite my ex-spouse's essential self. At first I tell him that I forgive him for being such a jerk. Gradually I'm coming to forgive myself and forgive him. Sometimes it may be about our children, other times about the financial stress I'm in, or still others about losing my best friend of so many years. I'm still working on it, but when I do it, I lose my vengeful feeling, the hurt goes floating by, and the hate is*

softened and released. There are times when I need to do this daily; others times it may be a week before I need to go back.

A wonderful side effect of this technique is that every time I do it there's a change in my life. Sometimes the changes come from my ex-spouse, but it also seems to open the door for others to help with just the right word or the hug that I've been missing.

How we respond to the obstacles that appear on our path is what matters. What we do is important, but the attitude with which we do it is more important. And we have a choice.

Stilling the Mind

Meditation practice is the most direct way to work on stilling the mind. There are a number of simple practices that anyone can do. If you have a busy schedule, you may not be able to set aside a lot of time, but if you can take five minutes a day, take five minutes. Five minutes every day is more useful than an hour once a month. You can train a puppy more readily if the training sessions happen every day.

It's helpful if you can create a special place for meditation. It doesn't need to be elaborate or require a lot of space; a corner of a room is fine. You can set it up in any way that feels right to you. Quiet is certainly helpful, but if that isn't possible, don't use it as an excuse not to practise. You can sit on a cushion or on a chair; sitting cross-legged doesn't automatically produce a still mind.

Some people, when asked to visualize something, immediately panic and say, "But I can't visualize; I'm not a visual kind of person." Don't worry. It doesn't really matter if you can visualize or not. Some people see images in their minds, and some experience life more through other channels. Perhaps you can feel or sense light, for example, more than you can see it. That's fine. If feeling rather than seeing the object of meditation is easier for you, then do that, but stick with it rather than switching back and forth; give your mind one less thing to think about.

Sit with your back straight, with your spine, neck, and head in a straight line. Because breath and mind are closely linked, stilling the breath helps to still the mind. First do the two breathing practices below, and then a meditation.

Breathing Practices (Pranayama)

In these practices breathe through your nostrils.

1. Inhale normally. Then exhale slowly and smoothly, trying to make the exhalation as long, slow, and subtle as possible, but without forcing the breath. Then inhale normally. The focus is on the exhalation, allowing the inhalation to come by itself. One round consists of a normal inhale and a long, slow exhale. Do ten rounds.

2. Exhale normally. Then inhale slowly and smoothly, trying to make the inhalation as long, smooth, and subtle as possible, again without forcing the breath. Then exhale normally. The attention in this exercise is on the inhalation, allowing the exhalation to come by itself. One round consists of a normal exhale and a long, slow inhale. Do ten rounds.

Meditation on the Breath

Sit comfortably in a meditation posture with your eyes closed. Breathe normally, visualizing the inhalation and exhalation of the breath. On the inhalation, the breath flows into the nostrils and down into the abdomen; the abdomen pushes out slightly. During the exhalation, the breath flows up from the abdomen, and out through the nostrils; the abdomen pulls in slightly. Concentrate on the movement of the breath. The breath should be relaxed, not forced. If your mind wanders, gently bring it back to the focus on the breath.

Meditation on Space

Sit comfortably in a meditation posture with your eyes closed. Bring your attention to your heart. Imagine there is endless space, like the vast, empty sky, in the region of your heart. Imagine that space spreading out, filling your whole body. The space can't be contained by any walls, even the walls of your own body. Imagine that your body is merging into infinite space. There are no barriers; there is only boundless space, and in that space there is only peace. Sit in that peace. If your mind wanders, gently bring it back to the peace in infinite space.

Meditation on the Heart Centre

Sit comfortably in a meditation posture with your eyes closed. Bring your attention to your heart. Imagine that in your heart there is a feeling of peace. You may see your heart filled with light or you may be aware of a feeling of contentment. Whatever else is happening in your life, this peaceful place in your heart is always there to return to. The light is forever shining, and love and peace are always there to welcome you. Sit in that peace. If your mind wanders, gently bring it back to the love and peace in your heart.

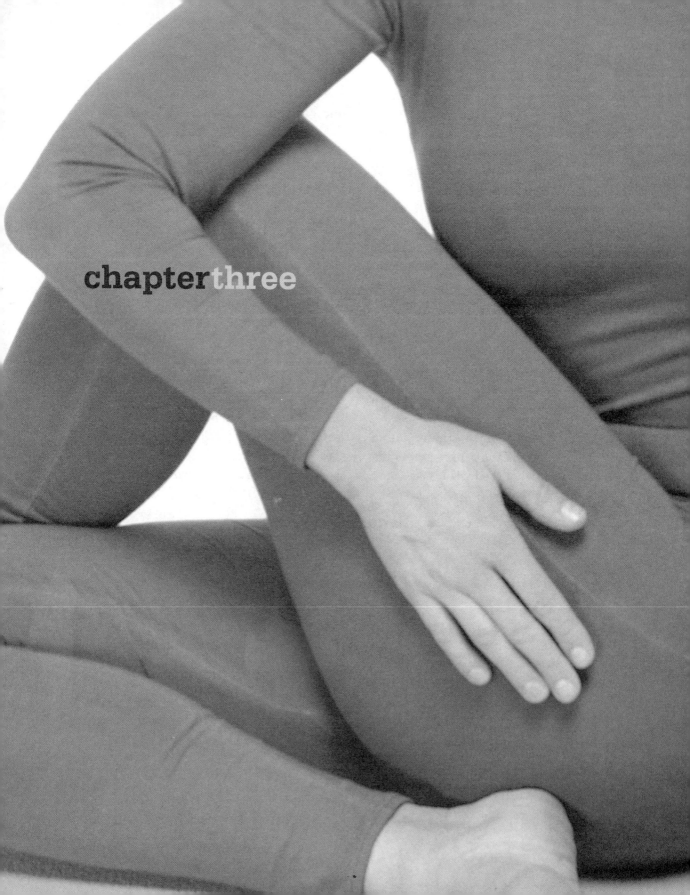

chapterthree

asanas:
the yoga postures

- What are Asanas?
- Desk Yoga Tension Tamers
- Asanas for the Back and Shoulders
- Yoga and Ayurveda
- Yoga and Devotion
- Restorative Yoga Practice

What Are Asanas?

Asanas are physical postures developed in ancient India by yoga practitioners who observed the natural movements of animals when they were sick. They saw that the sitting and standing postures of sick animals would change, and the sickness would be naturally cured.

With the aim of peace, yogis adapted those movements to benefit their own health and well-being, specifically to prepare the body to sit with ease for breathing practices (pranayama) and meditation. Asanas were developed that affect the internal organs, the glands and the nerves, and the muscular structure of the body.

Asanas are an important part of yoga practice. For the mind to be healthy, the body must be healthy. By teaching the body to be still and relaxed, we allow our mind to become still and peaceful; concentration and meditation then become possible.

In the modern world, asanas also give our bodies the strength and flexibility we need for the active lives we lead. Whether asanas are practised on their own, or combined with a practice of pranayama and meditation, we feel better, have more energy, and our minds are calmer as we perform the many tasks and duties of daily life.

How to Practise

In the practice of asana our aim is to unite body, mind, and breath. We practise to keep the body movement slow and thoughtful, the breath smooth, slow, and deep, and the mind concentrated.

Practise according to your own strength and flexibility, without forcing your body. Awareness, concentration, and effort are much more important than your ability to achieve a difficult pose. You'll find that as you continue to practise your body will naturally move more easily into the postures. You will become stronger and more flexible, your concentration will improve, and your mind will become calmer.

Warm-ups

It's important to warm up your body before asanas. Any exercises that increase circulation throughout the body may be done, or try the following routine:

- Shoulder Shrugs (page 152)
- Neck Warm-ups (page 153)
- Cat Flow Pose (page 158)
- Extended Child Pose (page 158)

Warm-ups are not necessary for Desk Yoga Tension Tamers or Restorative Yoga.

Guidelines for Asana Practice

- Wear comfortable, loose clothing. The models in the photographs are wearing clothing designed to show the details of each posture. You don't need special exercise clothes.
- Wait three hours after a big meal before practising, and after asanas wait 20 minutes before eating or bathing.
- Asana practice prepares the body to sit easily. In daily practice, however, it is better to do asanas after pranayama and meditation rather than before, since asanas stimulate the mind, a hindrance in meditation.
- Practise on a mat, to provide a soft surface and to protect you from the cold. Sticky yoga mats are ideal because they are non-slip; if you don't have a mat, then a blanket or a rug can work.
- Always warm up your body before doing asanas.
- Always breathe through your nostrils unless specified otherwise.
- Always do the Relaxation Pose for 5 to 10 minutes at the end of your asana practice time. After several strenuous asanas do the Relaxation Pose for 15 to 20 seconds.

About the Asanas in This Book

This chapter offers an introduction to practice through several asana sequences, each addressing a specific area or health concern.

The ancient Indian language of Sanskrit is the original and universal language of asana practice, and for this reason the Sanskrit name for each classical asana is included. The poses that are derived from, or simply in the style of, classical asanas have no Sanskrit name.

We hope you enjoy this taste of asana practice. If you find that you want to pursue further study, we suggest that you locate a yoga teacher in your area. In addition, there are many books offering an extensive study of asana practice. Refer to our suggested reading list on page 240.

Cautions

• Asana is a self-care practice. Please treat your body gently and mindfully, and allow yourself to progress in your own natural way. Your body is unique and your asana progress will also be unique to you.

• Do not do asanas if you have a fever.

• Do not do inverted poses during the first three days of menstruation, as they interrupt the natural outflow of blood.

• If you're pregnant or post-operative, have a physical handicap, diabetes, heart disease, high blood pressure, or any other serious disease, please seek the advice of an experienced yoga teacher and see your doctor before beginning an asana practice.

Tips to Assist Your Practice

• If you're feeling stiff, cold, and tense, try drinking a cup of hot ginger tea before your practice. Or oil your body with unrefined sesame oil, then wait 10 minutes and soak in a warm bath. You'll feel warmer and more relaxed for your asana practice.

• If you feel sluggish and lazy, drink a small cup of chai (recipe, page 43), wait 10 minutes, and then do asanas. If black tea isn't for you, try a cup of hot ginger tea.

To overcome resistance to practice, try the following:

• Start with your favourite poses or stretches.

• Commit to doing only five minutes and then see what happens.

• Jump-start your practice by going to a class.

• Experiment with different styles of asanas. You may need more heat, movement, and sweat, or more meditative yoga with slow, relaxing stretches and breath work.

relaxation pose
shavasana

Shavasana is traditionally known as the Corpse Pose because, when practised correctly, the body is perfectly still, the mind thoughtless.

We generally practise Shavasana for 15 to 20 seconds after each series or after several strenuous asanas. At the end of asana practice we practise Shavasana for 5 to 10 minutes. It can also be practised after pranayama and meditation.

The classic pose is done lying on your back as flat as you can possibly be. However, if needed, you can add a small pillow or folded blanket under your head to prevent strain on your neck. If your back is sensitive, a bolster or rolled-up blanket under your knees will take the strain off your lower back.

Letting go

To help yourself relax into Shavasana you can begin with the following exercise:

- Lie flat on the floor.
- Point your toes and then relax them.
- Tighten your legs, lift them a few inches off the floor for a moment or two, then drop your legs and let them relax.
- Tighten your bottom, lift your hips off the floor, lower them and relax.
- Raise your chest off the floor for a moment and then relax back to lying.
- Raise your arms about two inches off the floor, squeeze your hands into fists, stretch out your arms, stretch out your fingers, tighten everything and then relax your arms to the floor.
- Squeeze your shoulders toward your ears, pull them down toward your toes and relax them.
- Roll your head slowly from side to side, and come back to centre.
- Squeeze your face tight, tight, tight, and then relax your face.
- Open your eyes and mouth as wide as you can; stick out your tongue as far as you can and then relax.

Practise as follows:

1. Lie on your back on a mat or comfortable blanket with your feet 12 to 18 inches apart and your arms 6 to 12 inches away from your body with palms up (approximate measurements; be comfortable).

2. Notice your alignment; symmetry will help your relaxation.

3. Let your legs and feet roll out. Close your eyes, adding an eye pillow if you like.

4. Relax your body, letting it sink into the floor.

5. Practise a few rounds of conscious breathing (page 176), and then breathe naturally as you continue to relax more deeply into the pose.

6. When you're ready to come out of the pose, slowly open your eyes, bend your knees, and roll to one side to come up.

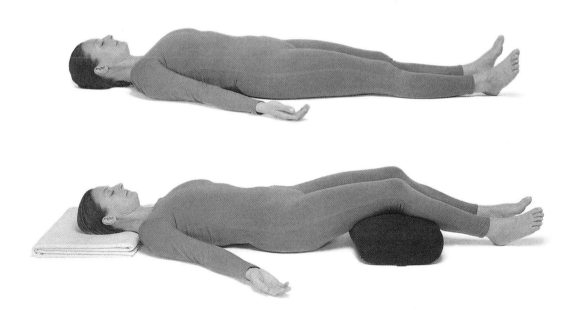

desk yoga tension tamers

How about a yoga break instead of a coffee break? Here is a series you can do at your desk or your kitchen table. Depending on how much time you have, do all of it or some of it; a little is better than none at all on a busy day.

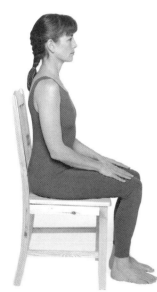

centring through the breath

1. Sit with a lifted spine, feet flat on the floor. Loosen belts and snug buttons.
2. Inhale through the nostrils, slowly and deeply into the lungs, expanding the abdomen, then up through the chest, filling your lungs completely.
3. Exhale through the nostrils—a long, smooth breath, gently drawing the navel in toward the spine at the end of the exhalation.
4. Repeat five times, relaxing into the sensation of your breath.

shoulder shrugs

1. Inhale, as you lift both shoulders up toward your ears. Exhale as you lower them back down.
2. Repeat several times.

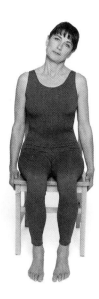

neck warm-ups

1. Sit with a lifted spine, arms loosely by your sides.

2. Exhale as you lower your left ear toward your shoulder; inhale as you lift your head back up to centre. Repeat on the other side. Do this two times.

3. Exhale as you lower your chin toward your chest. Inhale as you slowly roll your chin up toward your right shoulder; exhale as you roll it back down to centre. Repeat on the other side. Do this three times.

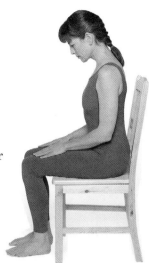

arm lifts

1. Inhale as you lift your arms out to the sides, shoulder height, palms up.

2. Exhale as you raise both arms above your head, interlace your fingers, and press palms toward the ceiling.

3. Stretch all the way up, through the sides of your torso, through arms and palms.

4. From this position, proceed to the next pose.

upper spine opener

1. Inhale as you draw your interlaced fingers in front of your heart.

2. Exhale as you turn your palms face out, lengthening your arms and palms away from the body and pressing your mid-upper spine back. Hold for two breaths.

3. Exhale as you draw your joined palms back to the heart area.

4. Repeat two times.

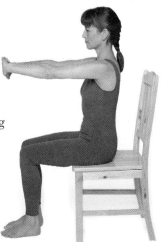

sitting spine tuck 'n' lift

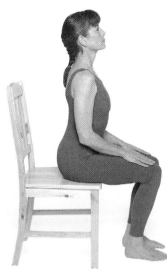

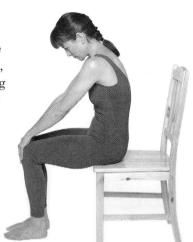

1. With your hands on your thighs, inhale as you draw your chest forward and up, creating an arch in the spine and tilting your pelvis forward. Allow your neck to lengthen.

2. Exhale and draw your shoulders forward as you release your spine, letting your pelvis rock back and your chin drop down.

3. Repeat these movements in a fluid, wave-like progression five times each.

side stretch

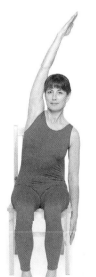

1. Sit with a lifted spine, feet parallel on the floor. With your left hand, hold onto the seat of the chair; inhale and raise your right arm straight up toward the ceiling.

2. Exhale as you lean to the left, keeping the lift and extension in the spine. Hold for three breaths; inhale as you come back to centre.

3. Exhale and relax. Repeat on the other side.

4. Do this two times.

ankle and hip openers

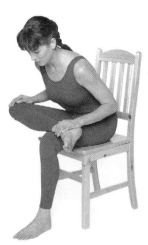

1. Extend both legs straight out in front of you, heels resting on the floor. Flex your feet and then point your toes. Repeat several times, breathing naturally.

2. Bend your left knee and rest the outside of your right ankle on your left thigh, close to the knee.

3. Inhale, then exhale as you move your abdomen forward toward your thighs, keeping the spine straight. Hold for several breaths, softening into the hip joint.

4. Inhale as you come up. Repeat on the other side.

knee to chest

1. Sit with a lifted spine and inhale as you lift your right knee up and interlace your fingers around the knee.

2. Exhale as you draw the knee to your chest. Hold for several breaths, breathing deeply into your abdomen and chest.

3. Release and repeat on other side.

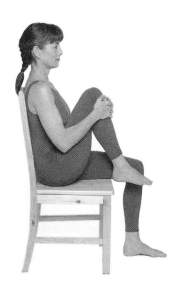

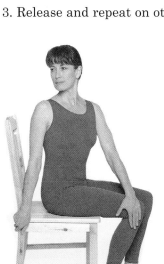

spinal twist

1. Place your feet flat on the floor, with the right foot slightly set back.

2. Place your right hand on the side of the chair and your left hand on the outside of your right thigh.

3. Inhale, lifting the spine up, and exhale as you twist to the right, using your arms only as a guide. Hold for five breaths, breathing into your abdomen and allowing your spine to lengthen as you rotate; release back to centre.

4. Repeat on the other side.

forward bend relaxation

1. Move your chair away from your desk about the length of your torso and head. Sit on the edge of the chair, spreading your knees hip width.

2. Cross your arms and bend forward at the hips, resting your forearms on the desk and your forehead on your arms.

3. Close your eyes, breathe naturally, and relax a little more deeply into each exhale. Follow the gentle rhythm of your breath until you feel ready to come up.

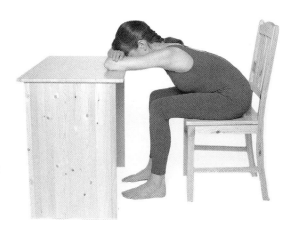

asanas for the back and shoulders

The spine is the core of our being. All asanas are primarily designed to move and affect the spine, releasing tension in the back and increasing the life force to the central nervous system. This series for the back and shoulders works well as a sequence, with one pose leading into another, or the poses can be done separately.

shoulder stretches using the yoga tie

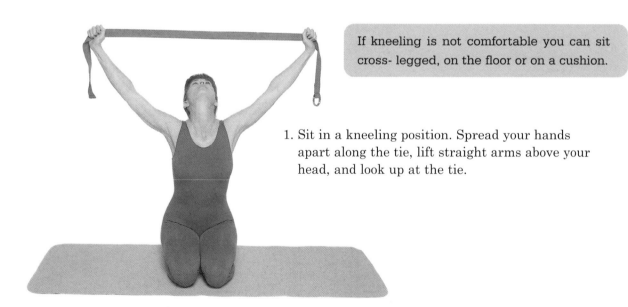

If kneeling is not comfortable you can sit cross-legged, on the floor or on a cushion.

1. Sit in a kneeling position. Spread your hands apart along the tie, lift straight arms above your head, and look up at the tie.

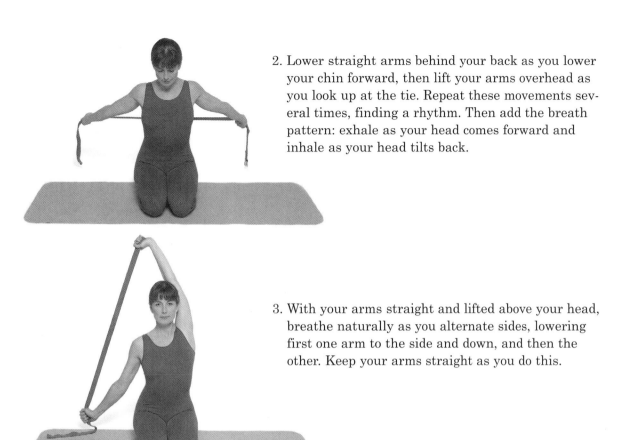

2. Lower straight arms behind your back as you lower your chin forward, then lift your arms overhead as you look up at the tie. Repeat these movements several times, finding a rhythm. Then add the breath pattern: exhale as your head comes forward and inhale as your head tilts back.

3. With your arms straight and lifted above your head, breathe naturally as you alternate sides, lowering first one arm to the side and down, and then the other. Keep your arms straight as you do this.

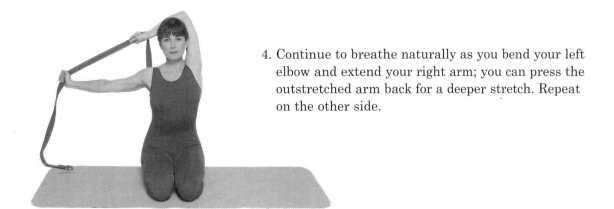

4. Continue to breathe naturally as you bend your left elbow and extend your right arm; you can press the outstretched arm back for a deeper stretch. Repeat on the other side.

extended child pose
balakasana variation

1. Extend both arms forward, bringing your chest to your thighs and resting your forehead on the mat.
2. Actively lengthen your arms forward. Breathe naturally.
3. Slowly draw yourself back up to sitting.

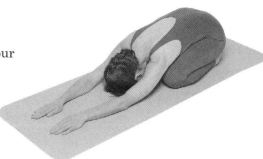

If this stretch is too intense try lifting your bottom in the air. If your head doesn't reach the mat, put a cushion under your head.

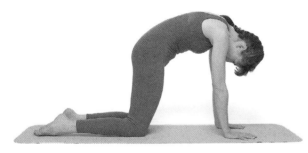

cat flow pose
vidalasana

1. Come onto your hands and knees, with hands under shoulders and knees under hips.
2. Inhale; exhale as you tuck your tailbone under and round the spine, pressing your chin toward your neck.
3. Inhale as you roll your tailbone up toward the ceiling, your belly moving toward the floor and your back arching.
4. Do several rounds at your own pace, feeling the whole length of the spine in your movements.

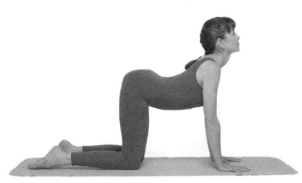

Allow your breath to become long and smooth; let the natural length of your breath guide the length of your movements.

extended child pose
balakasana variation

See previous page.

Remember to actively lengthen your arms forward and breathe naturally.

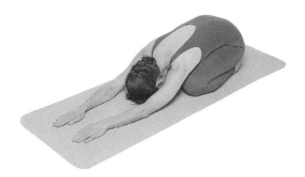

sunbird pose

1. Come up onto your hands and knees with hands under shoulders and knees under hips.
2. Breathe naturally as you lift your right leg, keeping it straight and parallel to the ground. Flex your foot and push out through the heel; keep your eyes looking down to lengthen the back of the neck.
3. Lower your leg and repeat on other side.

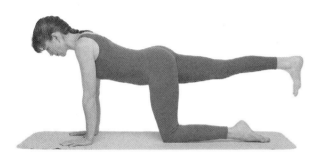

extended child pose with lifted arms
balakasana variation

1. Begin in Child Pose, arms by your sides with palms facing up.
2. Join your hands behind your back and lift your arms toward the ceiling, lifting only as high as you are comfortable. Breathe naturally.
3. Release back into the Child Pose.

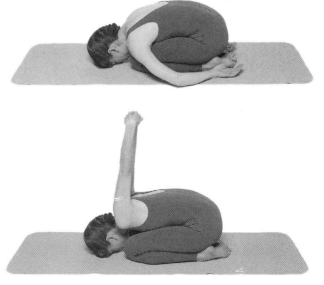

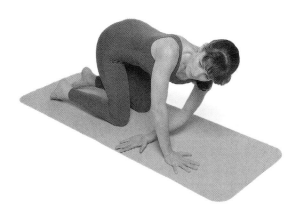

thread the needle

1. Come onto your hands and knees. Turn your left palm face up.

2. Breathe naturally as you extend your left arm diagonally to the right, coming down onto the upper arm and the side of your head.

3. Raise your right arm straight up and let the arm and shoulder roll back.

4. To come out of the pose, lower your right hand to the mat, under the shoulder, and press up to return to hands and knees.

5. Repeat on the other side.

For a more challenging twist, bend the elbow of the raised arm and rest the arm across your back.

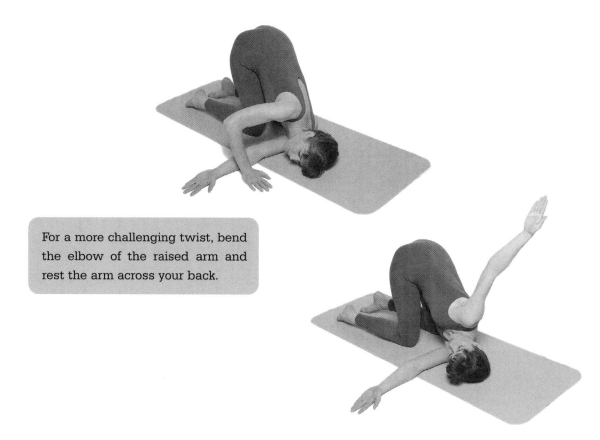

sphinx pose
variant of bhujangasana

1. Lie on your stomach, with your forehead on the mat and your arms extended forward, shoulder-width apart.

2. Lift your head and upper chest gently, breathing naturally.

3. Walk your hands in toward you so your elbows are under your shoulders.

4. Press down through forearms and shoulders, lifting your chest forward and up with your eyes looking forward. Breathe naturally.

5. Walk your arms back out, turn your head to one side, and relax.

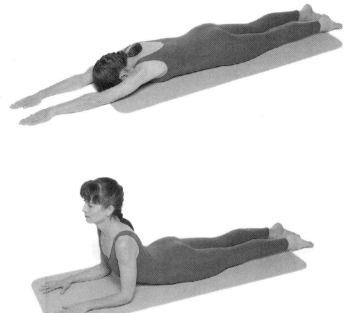

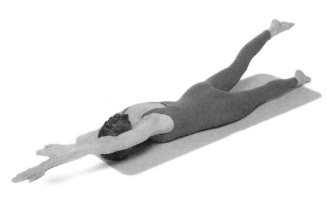

alternate limb lift

1. Lie on your stomach, with your forehead resting on the mat and your arms extended forward.

2. Inhale, lifting and lengthening your right leg with toes pointed. Breathe naturally as you hold this position.

3. With your forehead still on the mat, lift and extend your left arm out from the shoulder. Breathe naturally, as you continue to lengthen and lift both your leg and arm.

4. Slowly release your limbs to the ground, turn your head to one side, and relax.

5. Repeat on other side.

moving, reclining spinal twist

1. Roll onto your back with your knees bent close to your belly and your arms extended out from the shoulders, palms down for support. Exhale as you lower your legs to the right, all the way to the floor.

2. Breathing naturally, bring your left arm up and over to the right arm, stacking your two palms, both arms fully extended.

3. Move your left arm in a full circle along the floor, starting by a) moving over the head, then b) past the shoulder, c) over the hip, d) along the floor in front of you, and e) back to the palms-joined position.

4. To come out of the pose, bring your left arm back to the mat so that both arms are extended out from the shoulders; turn palms down, lift your knees, and roll onto your back.

5. Raise your knees toward your chest and wrap your arms around them. Inhale; exhale and press your knees into your chest for the Wind Release Pose. Inhale as you release the pressure. Do this two times.

6. Repeat on the other side.

• From the palms-joined position you can deepen the stretch by extending your right arm even further, past your left hand.

• You can also extend and lengthen both arms together, for a deep stretch through the mid thoracic spine.

1 and 4

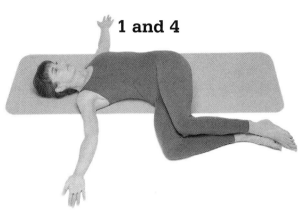

2 and 3e

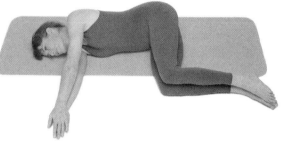

3a

3b

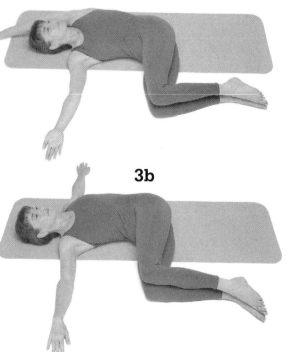

3c

3d

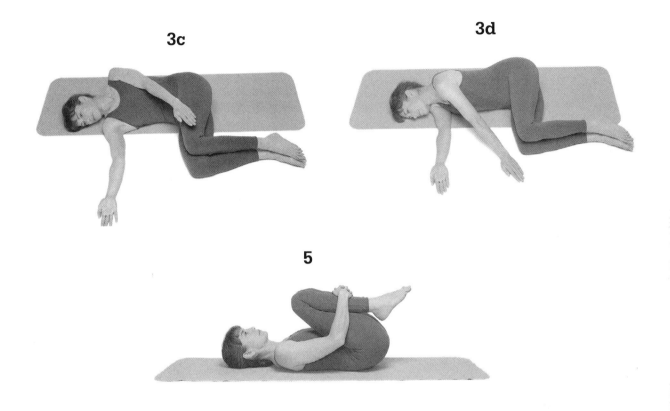

5

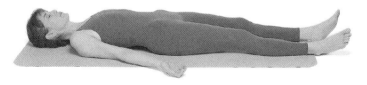

relaxation pose
shavasana

Relax in Shavasana until you are ready
to get up. Roll on your side to come out
of the pose.

yoga and ayurveda

After exploring the Ayurveda chapter you may have an understanding of your nature and imbalances according to Ayurveda. Perhaps you will be ready to design a fitness program to help balance your doshas.

You can choose from the following poses to add to your asana practice; there is one series to balance each dosha and one tridosha series, balanced for all doshas. You can make any routine tridosha by including balancing and relaxation poses for Vata, spinal twists and forward bends for Pitta, and backward bends for Kapha.

Remember to listen to your body as you practise. Pay attention to how you feel and whether you're getting the results you want. Remember that Ayurveda counts experience as important as theory.

Asanas to Balance Vata

tree pose
vrikshasana

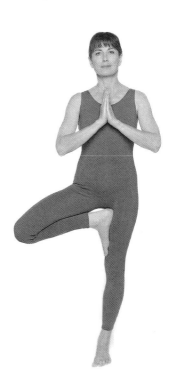

1. Stand with feet together. Raise your right foot and place the sole against the inside of your left thigh.
2. Place your hands in front of your chest with the palms together and fingers pointing upward. Fix your gaze on an object at eye level.
3. Breathing naturally, hold the pose for several breaths.
4. Lower your foot and repeat on other side.

In balancing poses always keep your gaze fixed on an object. This will help you keep your balance.

squat pose
upaveshasana

1. Stand with feet slightly apart. Exhale as you bend forward, bending your knees enough to bring your fingertips to the mat.

2. Inhale; exhale as you lift your heels off the mat and sit back on your heels with your weight on the balls of your feet.

3. Breathing naturally, place your palms together with fingertips pointing to your chin. Fix your gaze on a point on the ground about two feet in front of you. Hold the pose for several breaths.

4. To come out of the pose, lower your fingertips to the floor, bring your knees to the mat, release your toes, and sit back in a kneeling position.

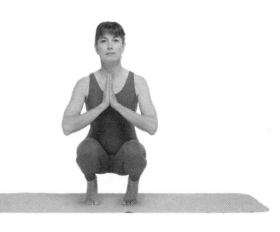

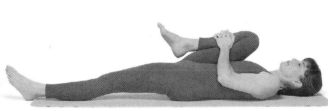

wind-release pose
pavana muktasana

1. Lie on your back. Inhale as you raise your right knee to your chest and clasp your hands together just below the knee.

2. Exhale as you press your leg as close to your chest as you can. Inhale as you release the pressure. Do this three times. Exhale as you lower your leg.

3. Repeat with the other leg, then with both legs.

relaxation pose
shavasana

Rest in Shavasana for 10 minutes or more.
Roll to your side to come out of the pose.

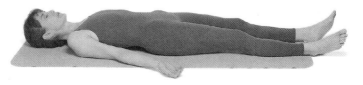

Asanas to Balance Pitta

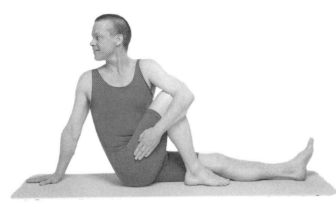

half spinal twist pose
ardha matsyendrasana

1. Sit with your left leg straight in front of you and your right leg bent so your foot is by your left thigh.
2. Place your right arm behind you with your hand on the mat. Place your left arm on the outside of your right thigh, with your inner elbow at the knee and your hand on the thigh.
3. Exhale as you lift your torso upward and gently twist your head and spine to the right, looking over your right shoulder as far as possible.
4. Breathing naturally, hold for several breaths. Exhale as you slowly untwist.
5. Repeat on the other side.

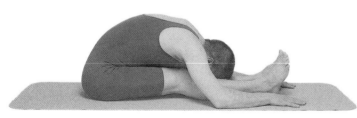

forward bend pose
pashchimottanasana

1. Sit on the mat with both legs extended forward.
2. Inhale and lengthen your back. Exhale as you bend forward from the hips, bringing your forehead as close to your knees as you can. Breathing naturally, hold the pose for several breaths, or for as long as you are comfortable.
3. Inhale as you return to sitting position.

full alligator pose
purna makarasana

1. Lie face down on the mat, arms by your sides.
2. Inhale as you raise your head, shoulders, chest, arms, and legs off the floor. You will be balanced on your abdomen. Keep your head straight, and lengthen the neck.
3. Breathe naturally and hold the pose for several breaths.
4. Exhale as you lower your body back to the mat.

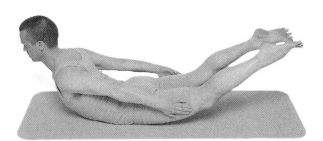

leg-hand lifting pose
uttana hasta padasana

1. Lie on your back. Inhale as you slowly lift your legs and torso. Hold your arms straight out in front of you and breathe naturally as you hold the pose for several breaths.
2. Exhale as you lower your body to the floor.

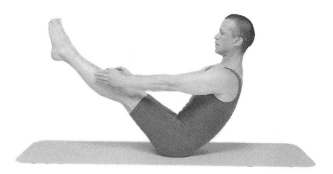

Asanas to Balance Kapha

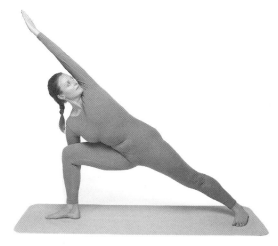

• To avoid knee injury, be sure that your knee doesn't extend beyond your ankle.
• If you are uncomfortable looking up at your hand, then look straight ahead.

angular pose
parshvakonasana

1. Stand on the mat with your legs apart about the width of one leg-length. Turn your right foot out 90 degrees and left foot in about 45 degrees. Lift your arms to shoulder height.

2. Exhale and slowly bend your right knee, lunging sideways until your knee is directly above your ankle and your right hand touches the floor on the outside of your foot. Your thigh will be parallel to the floor.

3. Stretch your left arm overhead, palm toward your head. Keeping your arm in line with your body, look up at your hand. Breathe naturally as you hold the pose for several breaths. Inhale as you slowly come up.

4. Repeat on the other side.

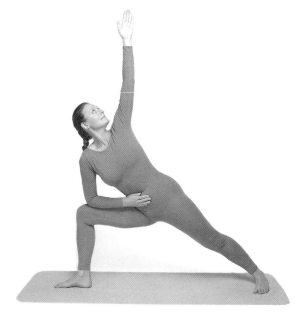

variation

Do this simplified variation if you can't reach the floor with your hand.

1. As above.

2. Exhale as you slowly bend your right knee, lunging sideways until your knee is directly above your ankle. Place your elbow on the inside of your knee; inhale and then exhale as you gently press back with your elbow to keep the knee directly over the ankle.

3. Stretch your left arm directly overhead, palm forward, and look up at your hand. Breathe naturally as you hold the pose for several breaths. Inhale as you slowly come up.

4. Repeat on the other side.

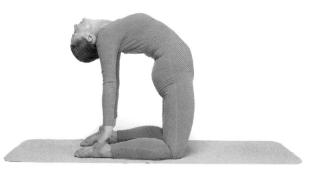

camel pose
ushtrasana

1. Sit on your heels, knees slightly apart. Reach back and grasp your heels with your hands.
2. Inhale as you push your bottom and abdomen forward, arching your back.
3. Breathe naturally as you hold the pose for several breaths. Exhale as you return to sitting on your heels.

For an easier way to get into this pose, kneel upright. Slowly exhale as you reach first one hand and then the other back to grasp your heels. Inhale as you press your bottom and abdomen forward.

bridge pose
setuasana

1. Lie on your back with your knees bent and your feet on the floor.
2. Lengthen your neck, keeping your throat soft and looking up at the ceiling.
3. Exhale as you press your feet and upper arms firmly into the floor and raise your pelvis. Lift only as high as you are comfortable; if your lift is high, place your hands on your hips to support the pelvis.
4. Breathe naturally and hold for several breaths.
5. Exhale as you roll your back down to the floor, first upper back, then lower back and pelvis.

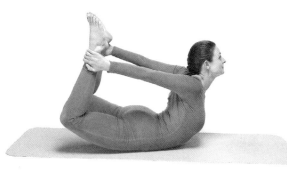

bow pose
dhanurasana

1. Lie face down on the mat. Bend your knees and reach back to hold ankles with your hands.
2. Inhale as you lift your head, chest, and thighs off the mat as high as you can, lengthening your neck.
3. Breathe naturally and hold for several breaths. Exhale as you slowly release and come down.

A Tridosha Series: The Shoulderstand Sequence

The four poses in this sequence make up a balanced routine for the doshas.
The poses are to be done in sequence, one moving right into the next.

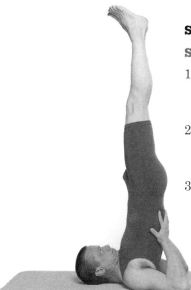

shoulderstand pose
sarvangasana

1. Lie flat on your back with your arms by your sides. Inhale slowly as you raise your legs so that they make a right angle with your body.

2. Support yourself with your arms and raise your body straight up on your shoulders. Your body now makes a right angle with your head.

3. Breathe naturally and balance on your shoulders for several breaths.

plow pose
halasana

1. From the Shoulderstand, exhale slowly as you lower your legs behind you, over your head. Keep your legs and arms straight and touch your toes to the floor.

2. Breathe naturally and hold the pose for several breaths.

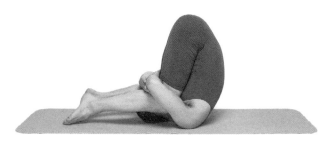

ear to knee pose
karna pidasana

1. From the Plow Pose, exhale slowly as you bend your legs, bringing your knees to your ears.

2. Breathing naturally, hold this pose for several breaths.

plow pose
halasana

1. Inhale as you extend your legs behind you to return to the Plow Pose, holding the pose for a few natural breaths

shoulderstand pose
sarvangasana

1. Inhale as you raise your body into the Shoulderstand, holding the pose for a few natural breaths.

2. Exhale as you slowly lower your body back down to a lying position.

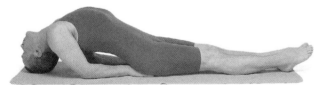

fish pose
matsyasana

1. Lie on your back with your arms by your sides. Inhale as you slowly arch your back so that the top of your head rests on the floor; raise your chest as high as you can.

2. Breathe naturally and hold the pose for several breaths.

3. To come out of the pose, exhale and press into the floor with your forearms. Lift your head up off the floor and slowly roll your spine back down to lie flat on the mat.

yoga and devotion

What is Devotional Yoga?

All of yoga has the aim of understanding ourselves, and of understanding that the ego of individuality is the greatest block to progressing on our chosen path to peace.

The practices of devotional (bhakti) yoga channel the ego in a way that draws us closer to God, Truth, Eternal Peace—many names are used to describe this state that we strive for. Those who practise Bhakti Yoga develop a relationship with the indwelling Spirit, one that is unique and personal.

The Forgiveness Asana Series unites asana with prayer. In this series we practise surrender to God, with outer movement expressing our inner faith and devotion. We offer our negative aspects, the egocentric traits that are obstacles to our self-development and spiritual growth, in order to reveal the universal and divine qualities within us.

Perhaps you are not comfortable with words like faith and devotion; you may be thinking that the practices of Bhakti Yoga are not for you. Yet this practice can be beneficial, regardless of your nature or your beliefs, if you think of it as an opportunity to forgive yourself.

On a psychological level, willingness to forgive implies openness to change. The ritual can help us embrace a state of mind that allows us to accept our own shortcomings and become open to the positive change we would like to see in ourselves.

The Forgiveness Asana Series
Ksama Prarthana Pranam

The nine asanas in this series form a flow of movement, connected at the beginning and end by mantra, in the form of prayer. One repetition of the series is as follows:

• Stand in Salutation Pose, stable, straight, and relaxed. Repeat the first mantra, asking for the removal of a particular negative aspect. (This mantra will change with each repetition of the series, each time asking for the removal of a different negative aspect.)
• Perform the series of nine asanas.
• After rising from the last pose back to Salutation Pose, repeat the final mantra, offering the asana to the Divine.

You can say each Sanskrit mantra followed by its English translation, or just say the English version if that is more comfortable for you.

There are 28 mantras for the beginning of the series and 28 repetitions of the series. When you have finished all the repetitions, practise the Relaxation Pose (page 150) for 10 minutes or more, until you feel rested and ready to get up.

Mantra for the Beginning of Each Series

1. *Namami tvam vasana-panayanaya.* I bow to Thee for removal of my worldly desires.

2. *Namami tvam krodha-panayanaya.* I bow to Thee for removal of my anger.

3. *Namami tvam bhaya-panayanaya.* I bow to Thee for removal of my fear.

4. *Namami tvam moha-panayanaya.* I bow to Thee for removal of my attachment.

5. *Namami tvam lobha-panayanaya.* I bow to Thee for removal of my greed.

6. *Namami tvam matsarya-panayanaya.* I bow to Thee for removal of my jealousy.

7. *Namami tvam krurata-panayanaya.* I bow to Thee for removal of my cruelty.

8. *Namami tvam bhrama-panayanaya.* I bow to Thee for removal of my delusion.

9. *Namami tvam asantosa-panayanaya.* I bow to Thee for removal of my discontentment.

10. *Namami tvam lolupata-panayanaya.* I bow to Thee for removal of my covetousness.

11. *Namami tvam satruta-panayanaya.* I bow to Thee for removal of my enmity.

12. *Namami tvam chala-panayanaya.* I bow to Thee for removal of my deceitfulness.

13. *Namami tvam alasya-panayanaya.* I bow to Thee for removal of my laziness.

14. *Namami tvam droha-panayanaya.* I bow to Thee for removal of my envy.

15. *Namami tvam avisvasa-panayanaya.* I bow to Thee for removal of my distrust.

16. *Namami tvam kapata-panayanaya.* I bow to Thee for removal of my deception.

17. *Namami tvam sandeha-panayanaya.* I bow to Thee for removal of my doubts.

18. *Namami tvam svartha-panayanaya.* I bow to Thee for removal of my selfishness.

19. *Namami tvam nirlajjata-panayanaya.* I bow to Thee for removal of my immodesty.

20. *Namami tvam akrtajnata-panayanaya.* I bow to Thee for removal of my ungratefulness.

21. *Namami tvam krpanata-panayanaya.* I bow to Thee for removal of my miserliness.

22. *Namami tvam apavitrata-panayanaya.* I bow to Thee for removal of my impurity.

23. *Namami tvam parigrahata-panayanaya.* I bow to Thee for removal of my possessiveness.

24. *Namami tvam duragrahata-panayanaya.* I bow to Thee for removal of my obstinacy.

25. *Namami tvam cancalata-panayanaya.* I bow to Thee for removal of my fickleness.

26. *Namami tvam dhurttata-panayanaya.* I bow to Thee for removal of my cunning.

27. *Namami tvam vyabhicara-panayanaya.* I bow to Thee for removal of my corruption.

28. *Namami tvam ahamkara-panayanaya.* I bow to Thee for removal of my egoism.

Mantra for the End of Each Series

Aham idam asanam brahmane arpayami.
I offer this asana to the Divine.

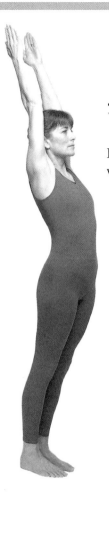

1. palm tree pose
tadasana

Inhale as you raise your arms straight up overhead, with palms facing each other.

2. toe touch pose
hasta padasana

Exhale as you bend forward with straight legs, as far as you're comfortable; if possible, touch your toes.

3. thunderbolt pose variation
vajrasana

Inhale as you bend your knees, sit on your heels, and bring your knees to the floor with your arms by your sides. Keep your toes curled so that the undersides are flat on the floor.

4. bowing pose
shashtanga pranam

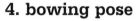

Exhale as you bring your palms forward onto the floor at arm's length and lower your body to touch six parts on the floor: palms, forehead, chest, stomach, knees, and toes. Your hands will be directly under your shoulders, your hips slightly raised.

5. cobra pose
bhujangasana

Inhale as you push up with your arms and lift your torso off the floor. Keep your abdomen on the floor and your toes curled so that they remain flat on the floor.

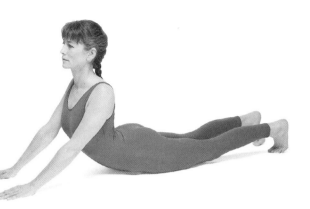

6. tortoise pose variation
kurmasana

Keeping your palms in the same position, exhale as you lift your body backward to rest your bottom on your heels and forehead on the floor.

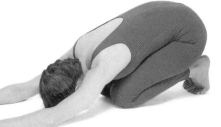

7. thunderbolt pose variation
vajrasana

Inhale as you lift your body to sit on your heels, with your arms by your sides as before.

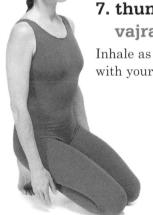

8. toe touch pose
hasta padasana

Exhale as you lift your bottom up, touching your toes.

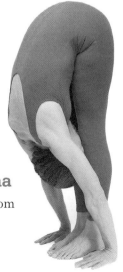

9. salutation pose
namaskarasana

Inhale as you rise to standing with your hands folded in front of your heart; keep them in this position as you end one set and begin another.

restorative yoga practice

What Is Restorative Yoga?

Restorative asanas are variations of traditional asanas, using supports to hold the body in position. Folded blankets, bolsters, and pillows are just a few of the props used to support the body in asanas that create profound relaxation and restoration. These poses allow the body to maintain asana postures with minimal muscular action, allowing more attention to the organs of the body, which then become more relaxed and deeply nourished by the breath.

Restorative yoga has its origins in the work of B.K.S. Iyengar, who experimented with supports, finding ways to enable students to practise without strain. He found that these modified classical asanas helped people to reduce stress and restore health at times when a classical asana practice was impossible due to weakness, illness, or injury.

Practise restorative poses any time your energy is low or you're feeling stressed from daily life; practise when you're recovering from illness or injury. Support yourself with restorative poses during the times you face any major life change or transition. These are the times when we don't have the strength for a regular asana practice and when we most need to be deeply nourished.

Supports

We use props to support the body and make it comfortable while holding the postures. We use blankets, bolsters, chairs, and the wall. We may also use tables, couches, cushions and pillows, belts or ties, and eye pillows.

Blankets can be folded or rolled, depending on the support needed. Belts or ties are used around the thighs to hold them in position without strain. An eye pillow is a relaxing addition to reclining poses. Made of cotton or silk, and filled with flaxseed (cooling and heavy) and lavender (harmonizing), these pillows are restful for the eyes. When the eyes are quiet, the mind more easily becomes quiet.

Most of what you need can be found around the house. Instructions are included here for making an eye pillow and improvising a bolster. See page 241 for information about buying yoga props.

Conscious Breathing

Conscious breathing is a method of centring through the use of the breath. It is deeply relaxing, and also helps us to keep our attention focused so that we don't fall asleep. When we are both relaxed and focused we can gently direct our breath to nourish the organs of the body.

We practise conscious breathing in reclining poses, that is, poses where we are lying on our backs. One round of conscious breathing is as follows:

• Inhale through the nostrils slowly and deeply, expanding your abdomen, filling your lower chest and then your upper chest, filling your lungs completely.

• Exhale through the nostrils, a long, smooth breath; feel your chest and then your abdomen gently drop as you empty your lungs completely.

• Now take several normal breaths, staying with the sensation of your breath.

In a reclining pose, practise up to 10 rounds of conscious breathing, and then breathe naturally during your remaining time in the pose.

Some Guidelines for Restorative Practice

In addition to the guidelines and cautions for asana practice given at the beginning of the chapter, the following guidelines are helpful for restorative asanas.

• Take out contact lenses before you begin.

• The poses are still, and your body will cool down, so wear warm and comfortable clothing. Be "cozy" for this nurturing and intuitive practice.

• When your props are set up and you go into the pose, check your comfort level. Rearrange if necessary, or try different props.

• Once you're comfortable in the pose, concentrate on "being," not doing. Just relax into the pose.

• Some poses may stimulate the kidneys, so responding to nature's call even during your practice is important.

BOLSTER

• A bolster can be easily improvised out of things you have in your home. Rolled up towels or blankets work well. Tie them with string or put elastic bands around them to hold them together. Towels and blankets can also be put in a pillowcase to make an effective bolster. Make your bolster about 6 inches high, 12 inches wide and 25 inches long.

EYE PILLOW

• To make an eye pillow, cut two pieces of cotton or silk fabric about 4 1/2 x 8 1/2 inches. Place them right sides together and stitch a half-inch seam around three sides, making a small bag. Turn the bag right side out and fill with about 1 cup of flaxseed and 1/2 cup of lavender. The bag should be about 2/3 full. Stitch the bag closed. Place it on your eyes when you are in a reclining pose or whenever you want to rest your eyes.

Restorative Asanas for Headache

The stress of our modern world often brings with it the tension that can cause a headache. Muscular tension and fatigue from bad postural habits will often increase the problem. Once we have a headache, we may increase the tension rather than releasing it because we tend to hold our breath when in pain.

The following asanas are designed to release the tension that underlies the headache and to open the chest for deeper breathing. Through regular yoga practice you'll likely find that you suffer from headaches less often.

supported bridge pose
setuasana

1. Place two bolsters end to end; sit astride, close to the middle.
2. Supporting yourself with your arms, lie down on the bolsters, slide your head, neck, and shoulders onto the mat, and stretch your legs along the length of the bolsters.
3. With your arms by your sides, relax in this pose for five to eight minutes. Begin with a few rounds of conscious breathing and then breathe naturally as you continue to rest in the pose.
4. To come out of the pose, bend your knees and place your feet on the floor on either side of the bolster. Raise your hips, move the bolster from under your torso, and rest your back on the mat.
5. Rest your legs over the back of the second bolster until you're ready to roll to one side and get up.

CAUTION
• Don't do this pose if you're pregnant, have serious back problems, or have an ulcer, hiatus hernia, detached retina, glaucoma, or head congestion (for example, a cold).

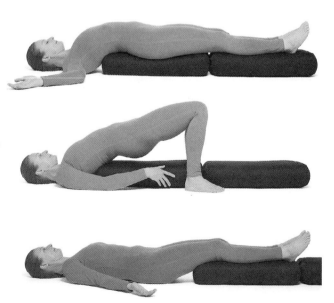

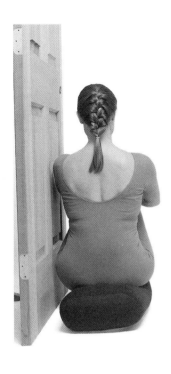

leg support inversion pose
viparita karani mudra

1. Place a bolster horizontally across the mat, about a fist-width away from the wall. Sit sideways on the bolster, close to the wall.

2. Supporting yourself with your arms, roll your back down to the mat and extend your legs up the wall. Your shoulders will be on the mat, the bolster under the sacrum. Lift your chest and roll your shoulder blades underneath you.

3. With your arms by your sides, relax in this pose for up to five to eight minutes. Work up to eight minutes gradually. Begin with a few rounds of conscious breathing and then breathe naturally as you continue to rest in the pose.

4. To come out of the pose, bend your knees toward your chest and roll over onto your side.

CAUTION

• Do not do while menstruating.

• Don't do this pose if you're pregnant, have severe back problems, or have an ulcer, hiatus hernia, detached retina, glaucoma, or head congestion (for example, a cold).

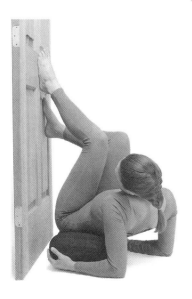

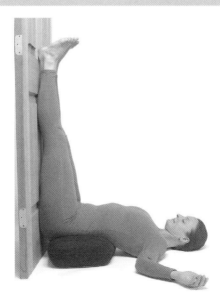

• If you have a long torso, and need more height to fully open your chest, place a folded blanket on top of the bolster.

variation

Do this simplified variation if you have tight hamstrings. It can also be done while menstruating.

1. Lie flat on the mat and extend your legs up the wall at an angle of about 45 degrees. A small support can be added under your head and neck.

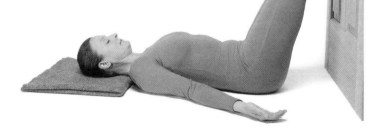

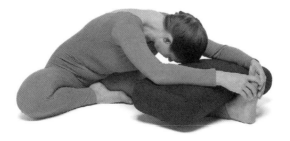

supported head to knee pose
janushirshasana

1. Sit with your left leg extended straight forward and your right knee bent to the side. Bring your heel close to the body, adding a support under the bent knee if needed. Place a bolster on the extended leg.

2. Inhale and lengthen your back; exhale as you bend forward from the hips and bring your forehead to rest on the bolster. Stay in the pose for two to three minutes. Inhale, come up, and repeat on the other side.

> • To assist the forward bend movement, sit on a cushion or a folded blanket to create an anterior tilt of the pelvis; this is very important if you have tight hamstrings or back problems.

supported forward bend pose
pashchimottanasana

1. Sit with both legs extended forward and a bolster across your legs.

2. Inhale and lengthen your back. Exhale as you bend forward from the hips, bringing your trunk onto your thighs and your head onto the bolster. Stay in the pose for two to three minutes. Inhale, come up, and repeat on the other side.

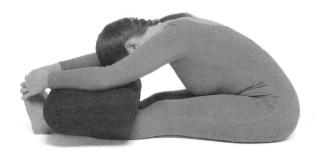

Forward bend movement comes from the hips and not from the waist. We "fold at the top of the legs."

relaxation pose
shavasana variation

Lie on your back with a bolster or folded blanket under the length of your spine. Adjust the height for comfort. Add support for your head and neck and rest your arms by your sides. Relax in this position for about 10 minutes, then roll onto your side to come up.

Restorative Asanas for Easier Breathing

An asana practice that develops increased lung capacity can be helpful for mild breathing difficulties caused, for example, by a cold, allergies, anxiety, or mild asthma. It also keeps the lungs healthy and flexible and increases the level of oxygen nourishing the body, which is important for overall health. The following asanas help you to gently open your chest and belly, allowing the breath to deepen. The reclining positions help to soothe the nerves and quiet the mind.

CAUTION
Don't do this pose if you have sore or injured knees.

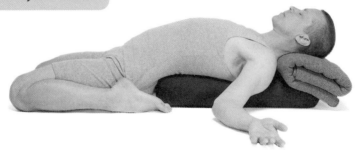

supported reclining hero pose
supta virasana

1. Kneel on the mat with your knees together. Separate your feet so that you sit between them.
2. Place a bolster behind you lengthwise, hold it against your lower back, and lie down on it. Place a pillow under your head and neck so that your chin is slightly lower than your eyes. Relax in this pose for three to five minutes. Begin with a few rounds of conscious breathing and then breathe naturally as you continue to rest in the pose.
3. To come out of the pose, come up onto your elbows, then lead with your chest as you push yourself up with your hands.

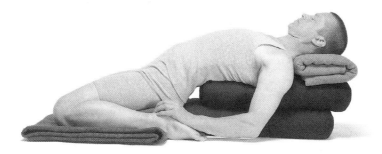

supported reclining hero variations

These variations are safe if you have sore or injured knees.

a) The pose can be done with added supports, building up the floor by sitting on a cushion; raising the level of the bolster with folded blankets. The supports can be as high as you need in order to take pressure off your knees and to give correct support to your back.

b) The pose can also be done with the legs straight out. This is the simplest way to make sure there is no stress on your knees.

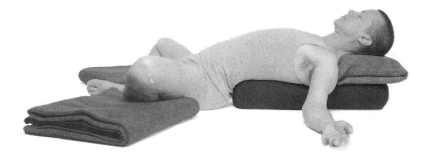

supported reclining nobility pose
supta bhadrasana

1. Sit on the mat with the heels and soles of your feet together. Bring your heels as close to your body as you comfortably can and place a support under each thigh.

2. Place a bolster lengthwise behind you, hold it against your lower back, and lie down on it. Place a pillow under your head and neck so that your chin is slightly lower than your eyes.

3. With your arms by your sides, relax into the pose for 5 to 15 minutes. Begin with a few rounds of conscious breathing and then breathe naturally as you continue to rest in the pose.

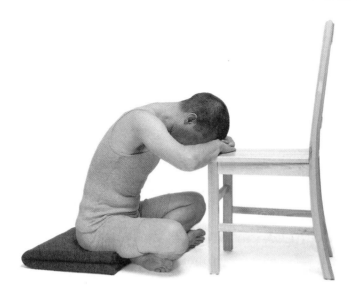

supported tailor pose
sukhasana

1. Sit on the edge of a blanket in front of a chair, with your ankles crossed. Bend from the hips and bring your head forward to the chair, resting your hands on the seat and your forehead on your hands. Breathe naturally in this pose for two to three minutes.

2. Change the cross and do the same on the other side.

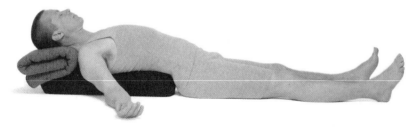

relaxation pose
shavasana variation

1. Lie on your back with a bolster or folded blanket under the length of your spine. Add support for your head and neck and rest your arms by your sides. Relax in this position for about 10 minutes, then roll onto your side to get up.

Restorative Asanas for Jet Lag

Flying can be a taxing experience on both body and mind. We sit in a confined space and breathe dry air. Our natural meal times are disturbed; in fact all our physical and mental rhythms are disturbed or suspended during travel time. The following asanas are designed to rest the legs, open the chest, ease the back, reduce fatigue, and soothe and quiet the mind.

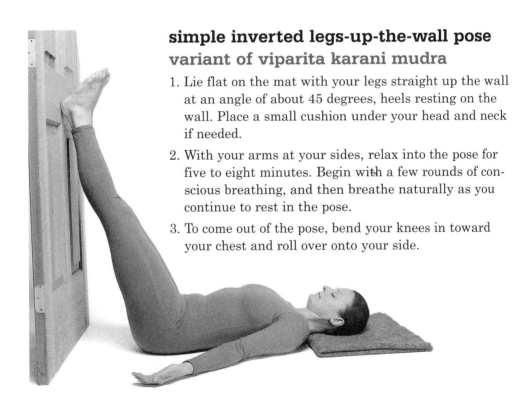

simple inverted legs-up-the-wall pose
variant of viparita karani mudra

1. Lie flat on the mat with your legs straight up the wall at an angle of about 45 degrees, heels resting on the wall. Place a small cushion under your head and neck if needed.

2. With your arms at your sides, relax into the pose for five to eight minutes. Begin with a few rounds of conscious breathing, and then breathe naturally as you continue to rest in the pose.

3. To come out of the pose, bend your knees in toward your chest and roll over onto your side.

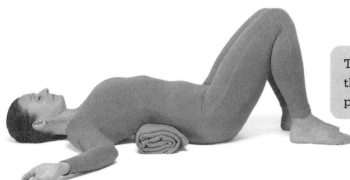

The support exaggerates the curve in the low back. Be sure to stay in this pose no longer than 3 minutes.

simple supported backbend

1. Place a small rolled-up blanket horizontally across the yoga mat. (The blanket should be no more than eight inches in diameter).

2. Lie down so that your head, neck, and shoulders are on the floor with the support under your lower back; keep your knees bent. Stay in the pose for up to three minutes, practising conscious breathing.

CAUTION

Don't do this pose if you're pregnant or have injury to the lower back.

alternate pose
supported reclining nobility pose
supta bhadrasana

This pose is less intense for the lower back.

See Asanas for Easier Breathing, page 182.

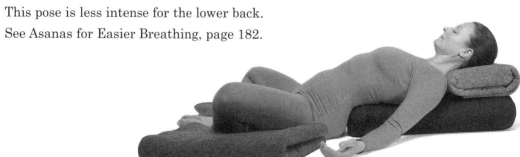

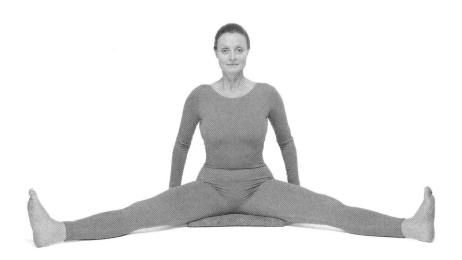

spread leg pose with supported forward bend
variant of upavishtha konasana

1. Sit on the edge of a folded blanket to get a forward tilt of the pelvis. Spread your legs out to the sides as far as is comfortable. Press your legs into the floor and press out through the heels. Stretch your spine up, lifting the crown of your head up to the sky.

2. a) If you're very flexible, place a bolster on the floor between your legs, bend at the hips, and bring your chest to the bolster. Put a blanket on top of the bolster if you need more height. Stay in the pose for three to five minutes.

    b) If you're less flexible, sit with your legs on either side of a chair. Bend at the hips and bring your forehead forward; rest your hands on the seat of the chair and your forehead on your hands. Hold the pose for three to five minutes.

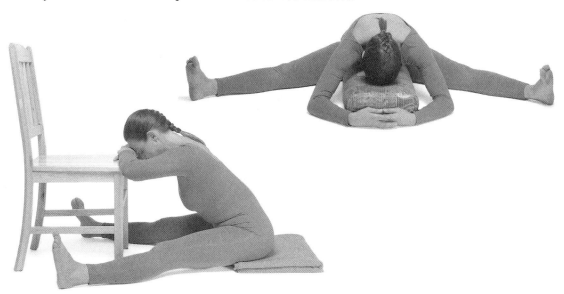

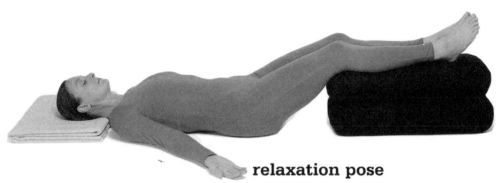

relaxation pose

shavasana variation

1. Lie flat on the mat with two bolsters supporting your knees, calves, and feet. A small pillow under your head and neck is optional. Rest with relaxed breathing for about 10 minutes, then roll on your side and come up.

> Tying a belt around your thighs can help to keep your legs from rolling sideways off the bolster.

> This can also be done with your legs on a couch or coffee table; just make sure that the angle between your calves and thighs is not less than 90 degrees.

Restorative Asanas for Menstruation

Asanas for menstruation are designed to be restful and ease discomfort in the belly and lower back. It's important to avoid strenuous and inverted postures at this time. A regular asana practice will often help to alleviate some of the more common complaints of the menstrual cycle, such as cramps, backache, and PMS. It can also help to regulate the cycle.

supported reclining hero pose
supta virasana

See Asanas for Easier Breathing, page 182.

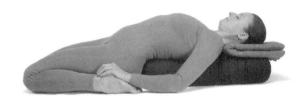

supported reclining nobility pose
supta bhadrasana

See Asanas for Easier Breathing, page 182.

spread leg pose
upavishtha konasana

1. Sit on the edge of a folded blanket to get a forward tilt of the pelvis. Spread your legs out to the sides as far as you're comfortable. Place your hands on the floor just behind your hips.

2. Keeping your legs straight, press the backs of your legs into the floor and press out through your heels. Press through your fingers and stretch your spine up, lifting your chest, and lifting the crown of your head up to the sky. Hold the pose for two to three minutes, breathing naturally.

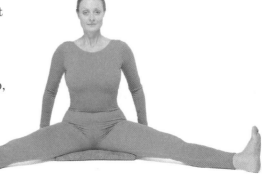

supported head to knee pose

janushirshasana

See Asanas for Headache, page 178.

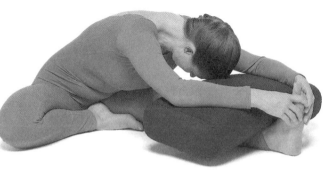

supported forward bend pose with folded leg

triang mukhaikapadasana

1. Sit on the edge of a folded blanket with your left leg extended forward and your right leg folded back. Place a bolster on your left leg and press that leg into the floor.

2. Inhale, lengthening your back. Exhale as you bend forward from the hips, bringing your trunk forward onto your thighs and your forehead onto the bolster. Hold the pose for one to two minutes.

3. Inhale, come up, and repeat on the other side.

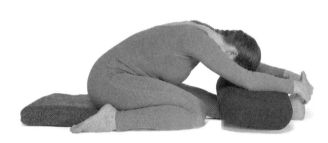

In the beginning you can let your folded knee move out to the side a little. Work toward keeping the thighs parallel. Contracting the left thigh will help to release your back for the forward movement.

supported forward bend pose
pashchimottanasana

See Asanas for Headache, page 178.

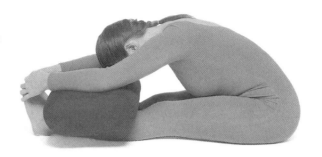

supported bridge pose
setuasana

See Asanas for Headache, page 178.

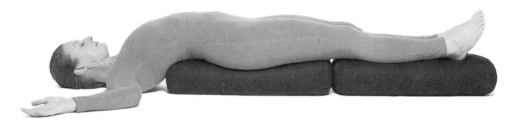

relaxation pose
shavasana

Rest in Shavasana for about 10 minutes, then roll to your side to come up. If your back or neck is feeling sensitive, add a bolster under your knees to flatten and release the lower back.

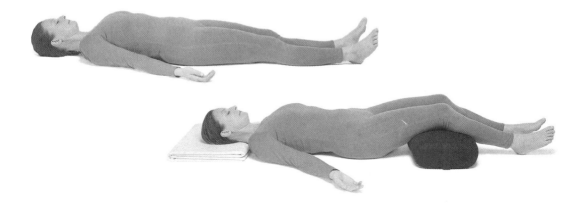

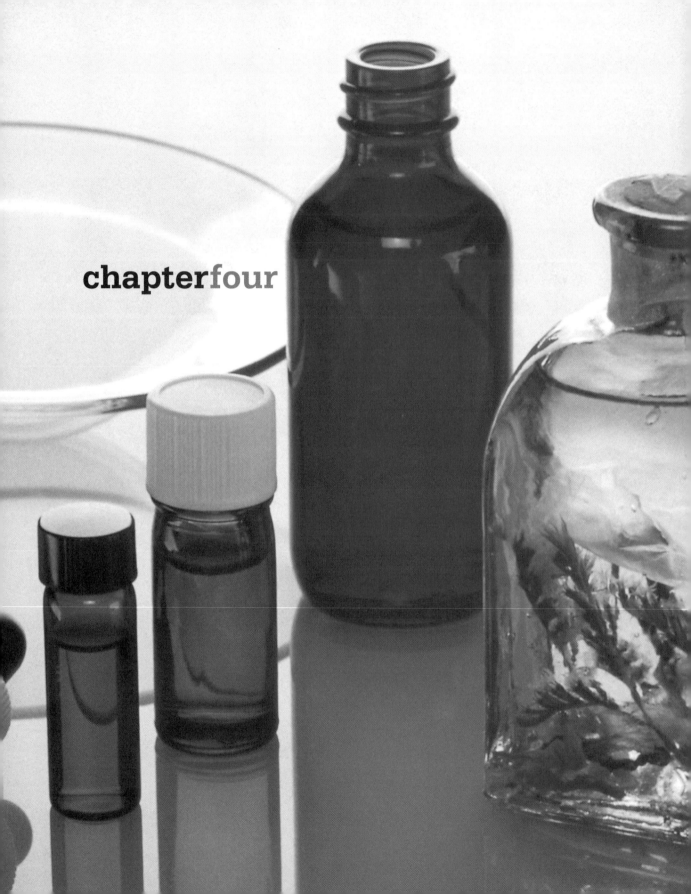

chapterfour

ayurveda:
one size does not fit all

What Is Ayurveda?

WE ALL WANT TO BE HEALTHY AND FIT, yet what works for one person doesn't always work for another. One person might not lose weight despite a strict diet and exercise program, while another person, eating constantly and hardly exercising, stays healthy and maintains a balanced weight. And what about the friend who feels invigorated on a hot summer day, while another is out of sorts after a short time in the heat? Apparently, one size does not fit all. What is the magic to health and fitness?

The answer, according to Ayurveda, is that we each have a unique body/mind nature. Our unique inherited constitution or "nature" determines what we look like, how we react emotionally, our interests, and even our health tendencies and risk factors for diseases. Some people are naturally lean and thin, others are stocky by nature, some are passionate, others calm, and some like to take charge and manage while others find it preferable and easier to carry out the ideas of others.

According to our inherited nature, different foods will nourish us or create health problems. Different diets, lifestyle, and fitness regimens will keep us healthy. Instead of one program to suit everybody, the Ayurvedic approach helps us design a unique individual wellness program to get the results we want.

Ayurveda is a 5,000-year-old science of life that originates, like yoga, from the ancient Vedas in India. It is the oldest continually practised holistic science and medical system in the world. In India, universities offer joint MD/Ayurvedic medical degrees, and many hospitals offer both Western and Ayurvedic treatment. In this chapter we explore the practical and preventive aspects of Ayurveda for the layperson.

According to Ayurveda, there is no single ideal health profile or baseline applicable to everyone. Rather, the health result we should each seek is to restore our original nature, which is experienced as our best weight, energy, strength, immune strength, personal power, passion, and balanced moods. Even when our aches and pains aren't detectable by Western diagnostics, Ayurveda says that this imbalance can be treated and our original nature restored.

The body/mind types, or natures, are explained by the tridosha theory. In Sanskrit, *tri* means three and *dosha* means fault, which is a dynamic, not static, state. According to this theory, life exists as a balance between three primary dynamic processes, or doshas. These processes exist in every cell. In each of us the three are in a unique balance or proportion that is natural to us—our "nature." This inherited nature includes health and disease tendencies.

What Is Your Nature?

Your nature is how your body/mind functions optimally. You experience your nature when you're happy, healthy, vital, and creative. It is your nature when your body's instinctive rhythms and responses and automatic activities keep you healthy.

From our parents and their parents we inherit a percentage of each dosha; this is our nature. Each of us has all three doshas in our nature; we couldn't survive without them. One dosha may predominate, two may be strong and one weaker, or all three may be equal.

If you have one predominant dosha, it will be easy to find yourself in the following descriptions of Vata, Pitta, and Kapha. If you have more than one primary dosha, you'll recognize aspects of yourself in more than one dosha description.

Vata

Vata is the process of movement and the force behind all movement in the body. Vata causes breathing, the beating of the heart, movement through the digestive tract, and blood and lymph circulation. It is the RNA and DNA in the cells, governing cellular movement.

The process is catabolic, using energy. As energy is used for movement, fats and liquids are depleted; someone who is constantly fidgeting, for example, will lose fat and muscle mass. Ayurveda would say the body becomes more Vata, more moving and dry. The main source (or seat) of Vata in the body is in the colon, where gases are absorbed and metabolic wastes are dried out and expelled.

Vata Nature

Those who have inherited more Vata are lean and thin, as movement uses energy and depletes fat stores. They may be very tall or very short. They like to move and may like to exercise, are often impulsive and may like change. Those with Vata nature are often artistic; they may be good dancers, performers, artists, inventors, theoretical thinkers, or idea people. They are usually better at initiating tasks than completing them, make friends quickly, and like to talk. Vata nature is spirited and inspiring.

Vata Out of Balance

When one's nature is Vata, one is prone to Vata imbalances such as disorders of movement and the nervous system, especially pain. Diseases resulting from Vata imbalances include arthritis, paralysis, diseases of the nervous system (such as Parkinson's and Alzheimer's), dryness (such as dry hair, dry skin, cough, or brittle bones) and unnatural rhythms (such as insomnia, indigestion, gas, or heart arrhythmia).

Under stress, emotional and psychological imbalances of Vata may manifest in worry, anxiety, fear, panic, schizophrenia, or excessive fantasy. Excessive accidents are a sign of Vata imbalance. In a fight or flight situation, Vata chooses flight.

Pitta

Pitta is the process of transforming matter into energy, creating heat. It is in the mitochondria in each cell. It is the metabolic process, present in the digestive enzymes as well as in the proteins of the body and in the red blood cells.

The seat (main source) of Pitta in the body is in the small intestines. This is where the liver, gall bladder, and intestinal secretions create the acidity of the body, necessary for cellular metabolism and formation of tissues.

Pitta is the acid chemistry in hormones and proteins. The fire of Pitta breaks apart matter and rebuilds cells; as it does this it analyzes and discriminates between nutrients and waste products. This discriminative process of Pitta is active in digestion, vision, and the intellect. In the form of a pH barrier, Pitta keeps the skin strong.

Pitta Nature

Those who inherit more Pitta are of moderate build and can generally eat a lot while staying the same weight throughout their lives. Their appetite is strong and digestion powerful. They may have a bit of a belly, which will possibly increase in middle age, and freckles or moles, red hair, early grey, or balding. They may have a higher body temperature than normal and tend to sweat more than average.

Those with Pitta nature have sharp, analytical minds. They like to be in control, and are good managers, organizers, and planners, as well as good teachers. They are good entrepreneurs who may like to run their own business in order to control their work schedule.

Those with Pitta nature have good gut feelings. They are passionate, sometimes even fanatical, and have strong willpower. They may feel they are always right, and often are, although a Pitta nature will try to avoid confrontation. They often like to push themselves to excel, meeting deadlines or juggling several things at once.

Pitta Out of Balance

When one's nature is Pitta, this dosha is more prone to go out of balance, often increasing the body's heat and acidity, which results in diseases of acidity and inflammation. All "-itis" and inflammation are Pitta imbalances.

Pitta physical imbalances include heart disease (inflammation or clogging of the arteries), ulcers, skin problems, fungus, intestinal worms, candida, belching and acid indigestion, liver and gall bladder problems, eye problems, sinus infections, and cancer. Addiction (to alcohol, drugs, sugar, or coffee, for example) often runs in Pitta families.

When stressed, Pitta nature tends to experience the emotions of anger, jealousy, rage, sadness, irritability, grief, blame, shame, or criticism.

Kapha

Kapha is the process that cools and supports the body. It is all liquids in the body and the process of liquification. It is the process of storing energy in matter as fats and liquids. It is anabolic (body building). Kapha, the bodily liquids and secretions (including lymph, fatty acids, blood plasma, and mucous), cool, insulate, and lubricate the body.

Water is the universal solvent, and nature provides an inner ocean of Kapha to carry, in dissolved form, all the nutrients and hormones needed by the body. The stomach is the seat of Kapha; all Kapha/liquids in the body originate in the stomach. The genito-urinary system is Kapha. Kapha is also in the cerebro-spinal fluids, in joint lubrication, and in the linings of the organs, eyes, nose, mouth, and lungs. In each cell it is the protoplasm. It provides the body's strength and maintains the body's integrity (immune response).

Kapha Nature

Those who have inherited more Kapha are squarely built, strong and sturdy, more naturally muscular, and slow and steady by nature. They have good long-term memory. They like routines rather than frequent change, and are good at completing tasks, although they may not like initiating them.

Those with Kapha nature are the ballast in a marriage or business, the glue that keeps things together. They tend to be compassionate, even-tempered, and emotionally stable. They keep friends (and enemies) for a long time and tend to stick with their job, mate, or project. They may not talk a lot, yet when they speak they have something to say that is important and well thought out.

Kapha Out of Balance

People who are predominantly Kapha by nature have good stamina and a strong immune system. Kapha is very slow to go out of balance, but when symptoms arise, the imbalance has been building for a long time and generally takes longer to correct.

Physically, Kapha imbalances result in colds, congestion, lack of movement (stiff or congested muscles or areas of the body, or laziness), contraction of muscles, excess water, excess weight, diabetes, low energy, and growths such as cysts and tumours. The first signs of Kapha indigestion are a feeling of fullness, stagnation, and no appetite at mealtime.

When stressed, Kapha emotional imbalances tend to manifest as an inability to make decisions or act, inability to make changes, numbness, denial, low energy, depression, or sluggishness.

The Dosha Questionnaire

The questionnaire that follows on the next page lists nature and imbalance characteristics for each dosha. It can help you to explore your tendencies when healthy as well as your tendencies when out of balance, or unhealthy.

Make a checkmark in each box that applies to you; if even one thing in a group applies, check it off. In the case of your nature, think back to when you were healthy and happiest and see which would apply to you then. You may check two answers to a question; however, if you check all three they will cancel each other out. If you aren't able to clarify by thinking of your happiest and healthiest time, just skip that question.

When you're done, total the checkmarks in each category and you'll have a starting point for understanding your nature and imbalances. By finding out which body/mind type you are, you can create a diet and fitness program that will restore your original vitality and nature.

Note: The Dosha Questionnaire is not meant to offer diagnosis of disease. For medical problems it's important to see your doctor.

PHYSICAL CHARACTERISTICS			VATA
Body Type	Nature		☐ Slim, wiry, thin muscled (stringy and hard muscles, not plump). Very tall or very short.
	Imbalance		☐ Dry skin. Too thin, can't put on weight. Arthritis. Cracking joints. Pain, any kind, anywhere.
Energy	Nature		☐ May vary—sometimes high, sometimes low, not consistent, level, or even.
	Imbalance		☐ Feels spacey. Low energy.
Digestion	Nature		☐ Prefers light foods. Prefers erratic mealtimes.
	Imbalance		☐ Food allergies. Gas. Indigestion.
Sleep	Nature		☐ Less, six hours or less.
	Imbalance		☐ Insomnia. Light sleeper—waking one or more times during the night.
Activity	Nature		☐ Likes to move and exercise a lot.
	Imbalance		☐ Fidgets, uncomfortable when still. Nervous. Tics. Pain, any kind, anywhere.
Evacuation	Nature		☐ Once a day, floats.
	Imbalance		☐ Constipation, hard, sinks.
MENTAL CHARACTERISTICS			**VATA**
Mind	Nature		☐ Quick mind. Fast comprehension.
	Imbalance		☐ Spacey, illogical. Talkative and skips subjects.
Work Habits	Nature		☐ Creative, has lots of ideas. Likes variety and change.
	Imbalance		☐ May not complete projects. Likes to initiate, but less follow-through.
Memory	Nature		☐ Good short-term memory.
	Imbalance		☐ Forgetful, spacey.
EMOTIONAL CHARACTERISTICS			**VATA**
Emotions	Nature		☐ Spirited. Enthusiastic.
	Imbalance		☐ Fearful, anxious. Variable.

Add up the checkmarks in each category and write the totals in the appropriate spaces in the chart opposite.

You can estimate the doshas as percentages; for example, 10 Vata, 5 Pita, and 5 Kapha would be 50% Vata, 25% Pitta, and 25% Kapha. This will give you a starting point as you explore the Ayurvedic tools for self-care that follow.

PITTA	KAPHA
☐ Moderate, soft muscled. Slight belly. Freckles, moles. Weight stays same.	☐ Sturdy, solid, muscular (often without exercise).
☐ Skin problems. Inflammation. Red or yellow complexion. Bloated belly. Heart problems. High blood pressure.	☐ Excess weight. Edema (water weight). Lipoma. Fatty deposits. Mucous congestion.
☐ High, passionate.	☐ Steady, level, usually doesn't push self.
☐ May push self, then burn out. High-energy times followed by low-energy times.	☐ Sluggish, hard to get started.
☐ Strong hunger.	☐ Slow. Eats less.
☐ Irritable or weak if eating is delayed. Acid indigestion. Belching.	☐ Loss of appetite. Weight gain.
☐ Moderate, seven to eight hours.	☐ Long, usually over eight hours.
☐ Acidity at night.	☐ Sleep apnea. Snoring.
☐ Short spurts, stops when hot and perspiring.	☐ Prefers very little.
☐ Overheats.	☐ Can't motivate self to exercise. Couch potato. Weight gain. Congestion.
☐ Once a day, floats.	☐ Once a day, floats.
☐ Diarrhea, loose, yellowish, sinks.	☐ Sluggish, may miss a day, sinks.

PITTA	KAPHA
☐ Sharp analytical mind. Strong "gut" feelings.	☐ Slow and steady. Thoughtful. Not talkative.
☐ Critical, judgmental of self and others.	☐ Sluggish. Lack of analytical ability.
☐ Good organizer, entrepreneur, teacher. Likes to be in control. Managerial, ambitious.	☐ Likes regularity. Slow and deliberate. Completes projects, has continuity.
☐ Control freak, does not delegate when appropriate. Abrupt. Perfectionist.	☐ Procrastinates. Less initiative.
☐ Quickly gets overall picture. Likes to learn.	☐ Good long-term memory. Takes time to memorize.
☐ Selective memory.	☐ Sluggish.

PITTA	KAPHA
☐ Passionate. Strong willpower.	☐ Compassionate.
☐ Anger, irritability. Jealousy.	☐ Attached. Depressed.

VATTA		PITTA		KAPHA	
Nature	Imbalance	Nature	Imbalance	Nature	Imbalance

Rebalancing the Doshas

Now that you have an understanding of your nature and your imbalances, you have a place to start in designing your own diet and fitness program.

The chart on the opposite page is preventative and restorative; it offers changes you can make to rebalance the doshas for better health. You can follow the advice for your primary dosha (the one with the most checkmarks) or your two primary doshas. You can also follow the advice for the dosha in which you are currently out of balance.

To chart your results, try keeping a journal, recording all the food you eat and your daily exercise. Note any signs of physical imbalance. Note also your energy level and moods—whether you feel energetic or tired, happy or irritable, even-tempered or volatile. After a week, then again after a month, look at your journal to see whether you're getting the results you want. If not, try something different. Ayurveda believes that the body wisdom, not a theory, should be the final word. Even Ayurvedic theory takes a back seat to experience!

If you find that you want help analyzing your doshas and planning a preventative and restorative program, an Ayurvedic practitioner can be a strong ally in self-care.
Note: The following dosha-rebalancing suggestions affect the underlying causes and not the allopathic diseases listed. The rebalancing chart is not meant to offer medical advice for treatment of disease; please see your doctor for medical problems.

The Food We Eat

The first tool for self-care is diet, which is literally at our fingertips. Ayurveda says you are what you digest, not you are what you eat. Even the healthiest foods can be improperly digested. Instead of adding needed nutrition to your body improper digestion creates toxins, called *ama* (literally, unripe).

Different body/mind types have different digestive tendencies. You may have noticed this when you eat the same foods as a friend does, and one of you is energized after the meal while the other is tired. To stay healthy, we should eat what we can properly digest, and avoid those foods that are hard to digest; this is not the same for everyone.

How Digestion Works

Each of us has our own natural rhythm of digestion according to our body/mind nature. According to Ayurveda, it takes between three and six hours to completely digest a meal. That means the digestive fire is "hot" every three hours, or every four, five, or six hours, at regular intervals.

The sign that the last meal has been digested is the sensation of hunger, proper hunger, felt physically in the belly. Real hunger is not a craving or a wish to avoid boredom; it is not a response to low blood sugar or due to addiction to candy or coffee. When we eat from this real hunger food generally tastes good and we feel satisfied and happy after the meal.

The Three Stages of Digestion

Before we discover our own natural times for eating, and why it's important to eat at specific times, it's helpful to understand the Ayurvedic view of digestion. According to Ayurveda, digestion occurs in three consecutive stages.

REBALANCING

Diet	**VATA**	Regular meals, every three to four hours. Warm, soupy, cooked foods like gingery vegetable soup with olive oil. More oils. Tastes: yes to sweet, sour, salty; no to pungent, bitter, astringent.
	PITTA	Regular meals, every four to five hours. Make sure you don't delay meals. Non-spicy, non-fried, non-acidic foods like cooked vegetables, dal, and rice. No oranges. Less salt. More protein if hunger is strong. Ghee for oil, in moderate amount. Tastes: yes to sweet, bitter, astringent; no to sour, salty, and pungent.
	KAPHA	Regular meals, every five to six hours, no meals after 6 p.m. Hot, cooked, spicy foods, not cold or heavy. Less milk, bread, pasta, sugar, desserts. Tastes: yes to pungent, bitter, astringent; no to sweet, sour, salty.
Lifestyle	**VATA**	Regularity, in bed by 10 p.m. Yoga, swimming, or fast walking, no running, don't over-exercise to an "exercise high." Oil massage, hot baths.
	PITTA	Keep the mind cool, become aware of, and express feelings and thoughts. Keep the body cool, stay away from heat. Moderate exercise, don't exercise when hungry. Moon baths.
	KAPHA	Exercise daily, increase activity. No day sleep. Keep warm, challenge yourself, communicate.
Herbs (Selected)	**VATA**	Triphala, haritaki, chavana, prash, drachsha, hingwastock, guggulu, ginger, cinnamon, cumin, fennel, ashwagandha.
	PITTA	Triphala, amla, red sandalwood, neem, shataveri, jetamansi, eclipta alba, drachsha, chavana prash, rose, red clover.
	KAPHA	Hingwastock, sitopaladi, pippli, guggulu, dashmula, cardamom, garlic, ginger, drachsha.
Dosha Balancing Asanas (Selected) (page 164)	**VATA**	Wind Release, Relaxation Pose, balancing poses like Tree, Squat.
	PITTA	Spinal twists, forward bends, backward bends like Alligator, Cobra (see Cobra in Forgiveness Series, page 175).
	KAPHA	Spinal twists, backward bending poses like Camel, Bridge, Bow. More aerobic asanas like the Sun Salutation.

In the first stage, Kapha dosha is active, liquefying the food, primarily in the stomach but also in the mouth and esophagus. Many vital elements are dissolved into the resulting liquid, nutrient fluid. This is the blood plasma, called rasa.

The rasa moves into the small intestines for the second stage of digestion. In this stage, Pitta dosha is active in breaking down proteins and fats and sugars through enzymes and digestive acids. The molecules broken apart by Pitta are absorbed through the intestinal walls and into the bloodstream, where they are transported to the entire body.

In the third stage Vata dosha is active in the colon, absorbing gases and excreting waste materials.

When We Snack

The three phases of digestion operate consecutively. If we snack continually, we are continually beginning the first process (Kapha) while further processes (Pitta and/or Vata) are still digesting the food we ate less than three hours ago. If we eat a snack just to "tide us over," we are actually upsetting our digestive process.

It's as if we threw a pebble into a pond, watched the rhythmic waves in concentric circles it creates, then immediately threw another pebble; the waves made by the second pebble create an interference pattern with the waves from the first pebble. Better to wait until the first pattern is complete before starting another pattern!

When We Skip Meals

Even more serious results occur from not eating often enough. Let's say it's 11 a.m.

and you're hungry (your natural rhythm is every three hours, and you ate breakfast at 8 a.m.). The phone rings or you have a deadline; you're so involved in what you're doing that you don't pay attention to your body's signals and you don't eat.

Perhaps half an hour (or three or four hours) later you find time to eat. Since you missed your body's natural digestive rhythm, you'll generally find that the hunger has disappeared. Sure, you can eat, but that strong hunger is gone and may not come back for several meals. Those digestive enzymes, that hot "fire" of the digestive soup, is no longer there.

The foods you then eat—though they may be healthy and Ayurvedic—won't be properly digested. You may feel tired after eating or experience gas, bloating, or belching. And what happened to those hot, acidic properties that were in your small intestines and stomach when you were hungry?

Pitta is used to break down food, and becomes neutralized in the process. If you don't eat when you're hungry, that Pitta, unable to be used for digestion, becomes toxic Pitta, and circulates in the bloodstream. It may accumulate and become lodged in a weak area of the body, later leading to disease.

Not eating when you're hungry upsets the digestive system. According to Ayurveda this creates toxins, not just from Pitta, but from all doshas. If we can't digest, we can't create proper cells. Systems start to malfunction, leading to disease if not corrected.

So the first step in Ayurvedic diet and nutrition is to discover your best times to eat and to eat at regular intervals. Finding and following your digestive rhythm is like priming the pump; once it gets started, the digestive fire improves and continues to come up at regular intervals.

Your Own Best Eating Times

There is no one proper time to eat for everyone; it depends on your digestive fire. You can find your natural digestive rhythm and best times to eat by noticing when you're hungry and eating at regular intervals.

As a general rule, if your main dosha is Vata, you'll probably feel hungry and need to eat every three to four hours (although you may find it difficult to regulate your eating times). If your nature is Vata/Pitta or Pitta/Vata, you may need to eat every three to four hours (and you may tend to use willpower to delay eating when it's not convenient). If you're primarily Pitta, you'll likely need to eat every four to five hours, Pitta/Kapha every four to six hours, and Kapha every five to six hours.

To find your natural times of eating, ask yourself when you feel hungry during the day. Start with breakfast—when do you first eat in the morning? Be sure to have actual food for breakfast—coffee, tea, water, or a smoothie will take away your appetite and smother your digestive fire. Hot, cooked, easy-to-digest foods, like soupy oatmeal or cream of wheat, are better in the morning, when digestion is slower and colder than later in the day.

After breakfast, when do you next feel hungry? If breakfast is at 8 a.m. and hunger comes again at 11 a.m., you may be ready for a snack or for lunch, depending on how hungry you are. In the middle of the day the body temperature and digestive fire are higher, so this is generally the best time to eat more proteins and fats, which require more digestive fire.

When do you next feel hungry? If you were hungry at 8 and 11 a.m., you'll probably find yourself hungry at 2 and 5 p.m., a three-hour cycle. Maybe you're more Kapha, and after eating at 8 a.m. you don't feel hungry until 2 p.m. Then that's the next time you should eat! You have a six-hour cycle.

Once you know your best times to eat, the next factor in good digestion is learning which foods are best for your nature. The best foods are those you can easily digest, and that don't imbalance your doshas.

Diet for Vata Nature or Imbalance

The diet to keep Vata balanced is one that keeps the body warm, rhythmic, and well lubricated, countering Vata's tendencies to coldness, irregularity, dryness, and too much or too little movement. The signs of improper digestion creating Vata imbalance are intestinal gas and a feeling of no movement in the digestive system.

Avoid: dry, raw, cold, carbonated, and yeasted foods such as popcorn, sprouts, rice crackers, chips, yeasted breads, raw foods, carbonated drinks, ice water, and colas. Avoid caffeine, smoking, drugs, corn, millet, potatoes, apples, and large beans like kidney, soy, or white beans (any beans that create gas). Avoid excessive fruits and sugars, hot spices, bitter greens, and astringent foods (like turmeric spice). Raw foods are considered cooling, and when taken exclusively can result in a spacey, ungrounded feeling in a Vata person; they can also contribute to serious constipation, especially when the diet has little oil.

Eat more: proteins; soupy foods cooked with oils; cooked vegetables; whole grains like basmati rice, oatmeal, cream of wheat and whole wheat tortillas; whole, organic milk; almonds; small beans like lentils or split mung beans; and spices like ginger, cumin, and basil. Olive oil, sesame oil, or ghee (clarified butter, see page 41) will help counteract the drying qualities of Vata and will create groundedness.

Diet for Pitta Nature or Imbalance

The diet to keep Pitta balanced is one that keeps the body cool (avoiding foods that heat it up) and the digestive process pH balanced. The first signs of Pitta digestive imbalance are yellow skin, belching, and acid indigestion. Above all, Pitta nature needs to eat when hungry—not delaying for even 20 minutes.

Avoid: spicy hot, sour, salty, or fried foods; yeasted foods like bread; citrus fruits; mangoes; red meats; aged cheeses; yogurt, fermented foods like beer and soy sauce; soy; chilies; tomatoes; eggplant; white potatoes; corn; peanuts; pistachios; excessive fats; cream; and sour cream.

Eat more: cooling foods like carbohydrates; cooked vegetables like broccoli, squash, okra, and sweet potatoes; sweet fruits like pears, peaches, and nectarines; whole milk; cooked rice cereal; cream of wheat; basmati rice; raisins; and small beans like lentils or split mung beans. For bread, try whole wheat tortillas with ghee. When hungry, eat more protein; when hunger is less, more carbohydrates. Ghee is considered the best oil for Pitta.

Diet for Kapha Nature or Imbalance

Kapha natures have a slower metabolism. They are "colder" and need to eat more hot-cooked, moderately spicy, and easy-to-digest foods. To add spice, ginger is recommended because it is the most balancing hot spice. The first signs of Kapha indigestion are a feeling of fullness, stagnation, and no appetite at mealtime.

Avoid: cold, heavy, sweet foods like ice cream, tofu, or baked potatoes with butter. Avoid cold foods and drinks, excessive raw foods, fruits, sour foods, salt, excessive liquids, sweets, and excessive carbohydrates. Avoid avocados, peanuts, excessive fats, fried foods, bananas, cheese, and milk (except in moderation). Avoid all oils except sesame, olive, and ghee in moderation.

Eat more: hot-cooked foods, small beans, soupy, easy-to-digest foods, ginger and moderate spices, cooked vegetables, almonds, and basmati rice. In moderation, Kapha can have spicy hot or sour foods like salsa, tomatoes, and fermented foods (Pitta-increasing foods) and light, raw foods like raw vegetables, sprouts, and rice crackers (Vata-increasing foods).

Balancing Diet

The best diet for good health is one that avoids all the foods that imbalance any dosha! This isn't as hard as you might think. It means focusing on easy-to-digest, cooked, warm, moderately spiced foods and avoiding acidic, hot spicy, salty, excessively sweet, sour, or astringent foods.

This balancing diet is full of proteins from red lentils, split mung beans, almonds, aduki beans, cottage cheese, or small amounts of mild cheese; carbohydrates from grains such as whole wheat tortillas, basmati rice, and cooked whole grains. It has cooked vegetables, milk, ghee, olive oil, and foods sweetened with small amounts of brown sugar (for Pitta), honey (for Kapha), or raw sugar (for Vata). It uses spices such as ginger, cumin, coriander, and turmeric to balance the doshas, while avoiding hot peppers and cayenne.

This diet avoids caffeine, chocolate, alcohol, garlic, onions, tomatoes, white potatoes, corn, cold foods and drinks, carbonated liquids, raw foods, and gas-producing foods such as cabbages or large beans.

Your Own Best Diet

A good way to determine your best diet is to experiment and record the results in a journal. For one week, eat the foods suggested by Ayurveda, at regular intervals when you're hungry. In your journal write the date, times of eating, and the foods you eat—all the foods, even one bite of something! Then, next to each meal or snack, record how you felt after eating it.

You may not notice anything until one to four hours after you've eaten. Note how your appetite was and whether your energy was good or low after eating. Notice if you had any sign of indigestion, or if you had a mood shift, a drop in energy, or any particular symptoms. If you felt vital and your moods and energy were level, then the foods and times of eating were right for you.

If you didn't feel vital, or you lost energy, either the foods or the times of eating weren't appropriate for your particular digestion. Try again with different foods or different times, always keeping the intervals between meals the same.

When Your Hunger Is Low

Low appetite is a sign of a weak digestive fire. Feed it the "'kindling" of easy-to-digest food and the fire will increase—if not in this meal then by the next one. Focus on soups or soupier foods and more carbohydrates and grains. Include lots of cooked vegetables. Sip hot water with (not before) a meal to help make it "soupier" and easier to digest. Eat less protein and less fats and oils, which require more digestive fire.

When Your Hunger Is Strong

If you have a strong appetite, throw a big log on the roaring fire! Focus more on proteins and fats, and eat lots of cooked vegetables. Eat fewer carbohydrates—too many carbohydrates will burn up too fast and this can cause an energy drop or "brain fog."

If you have extreme hunger because you waited too long to eat, your digestive fire will be weak and out of balance. Eat as if for low hunger.

Fitness and Lifestyle

Three people went to the gym. The Vata started running for an hour, even though his knees hurt; the Pitta was determined to push to a new personal record and was soon drowning in sweat, while the Kapha decided to go to the juice bar and have some food before getting started—if she got started at all.

These three people are choosing fitness programs that create imbalance in their constitution! We often do this. If we are Vata we choose things with more motion, so that we feel spacey, aggravate joints, and increase pain. If we are Pitta we use willpower to push through the body's resistance, increasing adrenaline and heat to excess, unbalancing Pitta. This is the Pitta tendency to "burn out." If we are Kapha, we may choose not to exercise at all, which makes our metabolism run slower and colder. We feel more sluggish and, if it's our tendency, weight and depression will increase.

To be fit we need to know our nature and our tendencies. Then, with full awareness, we need to find out what works for us. It may not be what we think, and it might be quite different from what works for our best friend, but if it brings results—health, energy, stamina, passion—Ayurveda says it is our proper regimen.

The following are some suggestions for fitness and lifestyle. If you don't feel more vital, your moods and energy more regular, and symptoms of imbalance reduced, then try the program for another dosha. Your own body will reveal the proper approach.

Vata Fitness

In general, Vata needs to slow down, and to eat and sleep on a regular schedule. Regular sleep and mealtimes help to bring up the digestive fire, which can be weak in Vata.

In fitness, more awareness of the body's limitations will improve results. Go into the discomfort zone but not into the pain zone; avoid pushing the body too far. In a workout, do more cycles and fewer repetitions. Running and aerobics are hard on the joints, a weak area in Vatas. Instead of running, try swimming, tai chi, yoga asanas, or aerobic fast walking, working up a sweat.

Heat is good for Vata, although the sauna can be too drying—try a sweat box, steam room, or hot tub to increase heat. Be sure to come out at the first moment of perspiration. According to Ayurveda, the proper amount of sweating is to just break a sweat and then come out of the heat. Sweating too long can cause overheating and decreased energy—you've been in the heat too long if you feel tired, spacey, dizzy, or rubbery afterwards.

Yoga postures to balance Vata are slow and stable, increasing heat as in the Iyengar style, or slow and grounded, inducing calm as in restorative yoga. Balancing asanas that are held for some time are good for Vata imbalances. The Wind Release Pose (page 165) and the Relaxation Pose (page 150)

Pitta Fitness

In general, Pitta needs to avoid getting too hot for too long. Stay out of the noonday sun; go on full-moon walks. Keep the head cool—when in a hot tub or sweat box keep your head out; in a sauna, wrap a cool, damp towel around your head. Overheating is particularly unbalancing to Pitta, affecting fertility, moods, heart, blood pressure, and the skin.

Never work out when you're hungry! Hunger brings up the heat and adrenaline in the body and so does exercise. The combination is a double whammy for Pitta, and can create such Pitta imbalances as anger and irritability, acid indigestion, and inflammation. Walking, swimming, and yoga asanas are the best exercise for Pitta.

To keep your heat down, drink enough water when thirsty. In a workout, do medium cycles and repetitions; note if your body is overheating and take a short break until it cools down. Pitta has a strong will—be careful you don't push too hard and cause an injury.

In doing yoga postures, be careful not to push the body beyond its limits, or to increase the body's heat, causing excess sweating. Asanas that flow from one to another, with enough rest poses, are best. Too slow may cool Pitta down unduly; too fast may heat Pitta up. Find your own balance in each class and asana. Postures that put pressure on the intestines, like the Spinal Twist (page 166), forward bends and backward bends are balancing to Pitta.

Kapha Fitness

Kapha natures generally hate to exercise. They would rather watch a movie or sit in a café, and yet they are the body/mind nature that needs exercise the most!

Running is less harmful to Kapha than to Vata or Pitta, because Kapha joints are well muscled and supported; however, since the "runner's high" can cause an energy drop, it's also not recommended for Kapha. Fast walking is preferable, and swimming is also good. In a workout, do more repetitions and fewer cycles. Kapha nature is the one that needs to push a little.

More aerobic yoga (like the Sun Salutation) that increases heat and raises the heart rate is good for Kapha. The Bridge and The Bow (page 169) help heat the body and reduce congestion in the lung area.

If you find that one of these regimens does not work for you, try one of the others. Your own body will tell you what does and doesn't work. Remember, your body wisdom is the final word.

Rejuvenation

Daily life in the 21st century is becoming more and more stressful. Unless we consciously simplify our lives, we tend to push ourselves to do more, sleep less, and work faster, rushing from task to task. We travel more to and from work, classes, or children's activities. We try to maintain more relationships than we have time for.

Due to this speed of living, and the stress we experience trying to cope with it, we may eat the wrong foods, skip meals, or overeat. Our digestive fire goes out of balance, our sleep is affected, and our moods fluctuate. We push ourselves beyond our limits and either burn out or feel sluggish, experience low energy, and feel depressed. Our body may respond with constipation, indigestion, or signs and symptoms of disease or premature aging.

According to Ayurveda, the body has the capacity to maintain health and restore balance. When we maintain the diet, lifestyle, activities, thoughts, emotions, and sleep that keep our doshas in balance, we stay healthy. Ojas (a substance and energy roughly equivalent to the Western immune system) maintains the integrity of each cell, organ, and tissue. Our body naturally eliminates the toxins that are created through improper digestion from the air, water, and foods.

When our natural healing systems are blocked (often, though not exclusively, through improper diet or lifestyle) the chronic improper functioning of the doshas results in an accumulation of toxins, which circulate and ultimately cause disease. These toxins are not considered disease by Western science until the fourth stage of disease according to Ayurveda. Because Ayurveda rec- ognizes signs of impending disease in very early stages of imbalance, it can focus on prevention when early symptoms arise.

Sometimes changing our diet and lifestyle is not enough to restore balance, and the toxins must be removed through rejuvenation techniques. According to Ayurveda, rejuvenation is the process of eliminating the toxins and restoring doshic balance. Because Vata increases naturally as we age (with excess Vata increasing the rate of aging and tendencies to disease) particular attention is paid to restoring the balance of Vata.

Ayurvedic Self-Massage

Ayurvedic massage is considered the first step in removing toxins from the body, and massage therapists are specially trained in this form of massage. In India, however, Ayurvedic massage is practised by everyone. Pregnant women are massaged, infants are massaged daily, and parents massage their children so that they will grow strong and healthy. Children massage old people, and men and women are massaged by the same sex. In this way Vata is kept in check, the immune system stays strong, and old age is healthy.

Ayurvedic self-massage can be done two or three times a week by a Vata body/mind type or when there is a Vata imbalance. For Pitta nature or imbalance, it can be done once or twice a week, less frequently in summer and not at all if there is too much heat in the body. For the Kapha nature or imbalance, it can be done once a week followed by dry brushing. To reduce or balance Vata, improve the immune system, and stay healthy, it should be scheduled regularly.

Ayurvedic Massage Oils

The use of warm oil is central to this body-work. It softens and loosens the toxins, lubricates the joints, reduces Vata imbalances, nourishes the nerves and brain, and calms and grounds the body/mind.

Ayurvedic massage and healing oils generally use sesame oil as a base; decoctions of various medicinal herbs are then boiled into the oils, making them potent with their medicinal properties, which the oil takes deep into the body. You can use plain, unrefined, unroasted sesame oil for your massage, or see page 241 under "Ayurveda Product Sources" for information about where to purchase oils with medicinal herbs. Here are some examples of massage oils for the doshas:

Vata: sesame oil, dashmula oil, mahanara-yana oil, garlic/sesame oil
Pitta: sesame oil, sandalwood oil, turmeric ghee, almond oil
Kapha: sesame oil, garlic/sesame oil, castor/dashmula oil, mustard oil

The Importance of Heat

Heat is also important in the Ayurvedic massage. The oils are heated, and the benefits of the massage are increased when followed by a hot bath, shower, or sauna. The use of heat reduces Vata imbalances. It increases the movement of toxins from deeper tissues in the body into the central digestive canal, and helps to burn up toxins and activate the body's natural toxin-destroying capacities.

The Self-Massage Technique

Although this massage can be done in as little as five minutes, it's best if you find a time when you don't have to rush. If time is short you can use the oil at room temperature instead of heating it; it will warm up when you apply it to your body. Whether it's done quickly or slowly, with hot or room-temperature oil, the massage will have a beneficial effect.

The general technique is to use your palms to massage around each joint in a circle, and use both palms and fingers to massage up and down the long bones of the legs or arms. Friction increases body heat and helps the oil to be absorbed; press hard enough to create friction but not so hard as to create pain. As oil is absorbed, add more oil. When the massage is done your body should feel slippery; the more oil your body absorbs, the more Vata is reduced.

● Begin by choosing your oil. Heat it, if you have time, until it is almost, but not quite, too hot to hold in your hand. To warm it, put the oil in a jar or a plastic squeeze bottle, place it in a pan with about two inches of water, and heat it on the stove top.

● Put one leg on the edge of the bathtub or sink. Massage each toe joint, massage up and down the top of the foot and the arch, and then circle around the ankles with the palms of your hands. Continually adding oil as needed, massage up and down the lower leg, circle around the knees, and then up and down the thighs. Do the other leg in the same way.

● Now put the palms of your hands on your hip joints and move your hands in a small circle, creating friction and heat in your hips. Massage the stomach in a circle: down the left side, across the bottom, up the right side, across the top of the stomach, then down the left side again, several times. Massage the buttocks, lower back, then up and down the sides of the ribcage.

● Massage one hand, circling the finger joints, circling the wrist, massaging up and down the lower arm, circling the elbow, massaging up and down the upper arm, then massaging in a circle on the shoulder joint. Do the other arm the same way.

● Oil and massage the neck, up and down, on all sides. Then do your face, paying attention to the sinuses. Massage the ears, including the insides, the head, and the hair. At this point your entire body has been oiled and massaged and you should feel your circulation increased, your energy improved, and your body waking up.

● Now go into a bath, shower, or sauna that is hot, but not too hot (warm if you're Pitta). The heat will allow the oil to be further absorbed into the bloodstream. You can use soap if you like, although it's preferable to use no soap, or use an Ayurvedic herbal scrub. (Most of the oil will not end up in your bathtub or shower, as it will be absorbed into the body.)

With proper heating your body will feel light and energetic; with over-heating you'll feel tired, light-headed, or sluggish. To prevent over-heating, come out of the heat as soon as you break a sweat or feel uncomfortably hot. Keeping your head cool can help prevent over-heating—in the shower or bath keep it out of the heat, in the sauna wrap it in a cool, wet towel.

Note: Avoid the sauna if you have your period, high blood pressure, heart problems, a tendency to dizziness, or if you're trying to get pregnant. Both Ayurveda and Western medicine have determined that fertility is decreased (in both men and women) with too much heat exposure. Even hot baths and hot tubs are not recommended if you want to get pregnant.

Ayurvedic Cleansing

The second step in removing toxins is cleansing. Pancha Karma is the Ayurvedic cleansing program said to have miraculous effects in reversing diseases, eliminating symptoms, and restoring vitality, energy, and mobility, even in severe cases. This is a powerful tool for regaining health, administered under the supervision of an Ayurvedic practitioner.

A simple three-day self-cleanse, however, is something you can safely undertake on your own. While not a replacement for Pancha Karma, you can expect wonderful results from a simple cleanse. You'll feel lighter, happier, more energetic, more grounded, with Vata symptoms reduced, digestion and elimination improved, and sleep sounder.

When preparing to do a self-cleanse, first ask yourself if you've undertaken a proper Ayurvedic rebalancing program with diet and lifestyle changes. A good pre-cleanse program is a balancing diet for two to four weeks (see page 200). If you haven't balanced your diet and lifestyle, a simple cleanse won't be as effective. Ideally, you'll have three days of rest and relaxation while doing the program, a break from the usual activities of your life.

Note: Don't do the self-cleanse if you're pregnant, have high blood pressure, severe constipation, or heart irregularities. If you have any serious disease, consult your doctor before beginning a cleanse.

The Three-Day Self-Cleanse

- For three nights, beginning the night before your three-day cleanse, take 1–2 teaspoons Triphala one hour before bed. Triphala is a gentle lower-abdominal cleanser, an herbal formula that is balancing to all three doshas.

- During the three-day cleanse, eat at regular intervals depending on hunger. At each meal, eat until you are two-thirds full; do not under- or over-eat.

- For breakfast each day prepare cooked, hot, soupy oatmeal, cream of wheat, or other grain, with milk or soymilk and honey for Kapha, brown sugar for Pitta, or raw sugar for Vata.

- For other meals eat only freshly cooked, warm kitcheree (recipe, page 42) with extra ghee (recipe, page 41) and vegetables.

- Each day give yourself an Ayurvedic Self-Massage with warm oil, followed by a bath, shower, or sauna.

- Fill your days with spiritual or inspirational reading, easy walks, gentle yoga, journalling, and deep resting. No appointments, meetings, or expectations during these three days. The journey is inward, increasing awareness of your own body/mind nature.

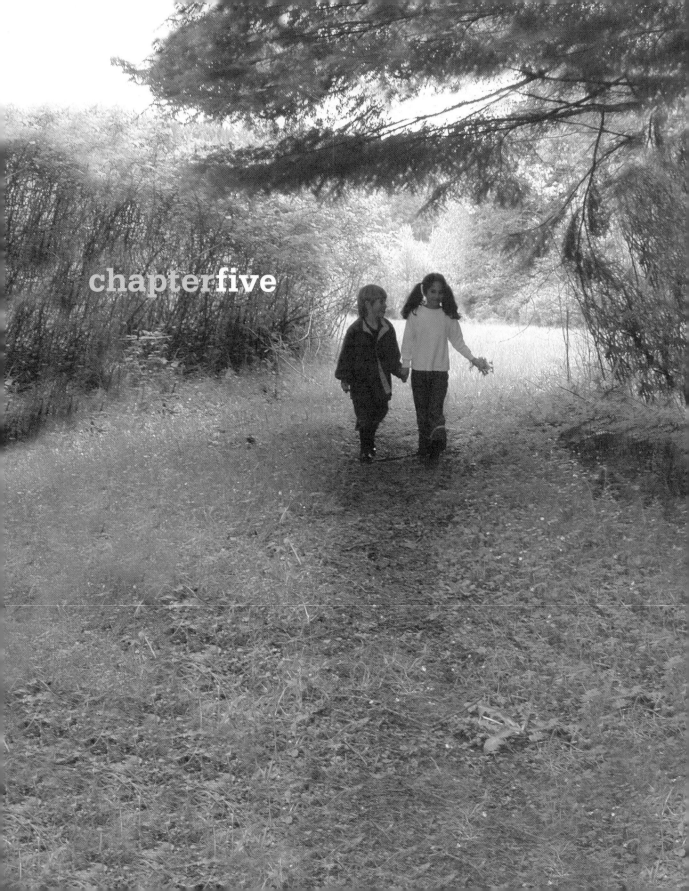

chapter**five**

in the spirit of play:
activities for fun and self-discovery

What Is Play?

WHEN WE WATCH CHILDREN PLAY, WE SEE THE CREATIVE, open-hearted, and spontaneous expression of who they are. Their play is without inhibition—they throw themselves into it with joy, exploring themselves, their relationships with others, and how the world works. And they have fun.

In this chapter we offer activities for creative self-expression, an opportunity for you to explore with the same kind of open-hearted spontaneity. Some activities are purely for fun; others are for reflection and self-discovery. The chapter opens with the making of a personal altar because we think that sacred space is a support and a comfort during self-exploration. The chapter closes with the Fragrant Flower Facial because it's both fun and nourishing.

About the Activities

There is no right or wrong way to do any of these activities. If you find you want to do something differently from the way we've suggested, then go with it. Your intuition is your best guide.

Remember that this is about expressing yourself, not about making art. Let your work tell you how it wants to be—assume nothing, not even that you know what you're creating. When it's done let your work tell you what it is.

We've included several collage projects because they're fun and easy to do. If you feel self-conscious about making art, this is a good place to begin. If you think back to kindergarten, you'll realize that you already know how to do this cut-and-paste activity.

You'll sometimes be asked to relax your body and quiet your mind, to help get the busy mind out of the way so the creative mind can "come out to play." Try the Relaxation Pose (page 150) to help you relax. You can practise conscious breathing (page 176) or simply notice your breath, watching as it goes in and out, in and out, gradually slowing as your relaxation deepens.

To do some of these activities with a friend can be a meaningful way to spend time together. It also allows you to talk together afterward about what you've learned, which can help to make new insights firm in your mind. Writing is another good way to fix a new awareness.

What You Need for Art Activities

Along with the instructions for each activity is a list of what you need. Some things you'll have around the house; others you can pur-chase or borrow. Most supplies can be found in hobby shops, art supply stores, and sometimes drugstores or hardware stores. Here is helpful information about some of the supplies you'll need:

• For drawing and colouring we like oil pastels or felt pens—they have strong, vibrant colours.

• Acrylic paints come in tubes or plastic jars.

• Use tempera paints for painting on paper. They come in tubes, plastic jars, or in paint sets similar to children's watercolour sets.

• Face paints come in pencils that you dip in water; they also come in paint sets like the tempera paints.

• When you buy paints, ask what kind of brush or brushes you need for the activity you plan. If you buy a paint set you'll probably need a better quality brush than the one that comes with it. For face painting, get a brush that will come to a point for detail work.

• Use white glue for gluing paper.

• You can usually get a small hot-glue gun at a hardware store or hobby shop (be sure to get the glue sticks that go in the gun).

your personal altar

TYPE OF ACTIVITY: SPIRITUAL, NURTURING

Your personal altar is an expression of your inner self, and so each one is as unique as the person who makes it. An altar may be religious, or it may be the altar of your heart—what's important is that you are creating your personal sacred space. Your altar might be on a table, a shelf, or a windowsill; its purpose is to give you a quiet place to be with yourself. Use it for prayer and meditation, inspirational reading, reflection, and journal writing—or just sit quietly, pause, and let the demands of daily life fall away.

How to Make Your Altar

1. Select a place that can be just yours, with room enough for a small table and a cushion or a chair to sit on. If you don't have a private spot choose the corner of a room or even a corner of your desk. Collect images and objects that are meaningful to you or that inspire you, and arrange them on your altar in a way that pleases you.

2. Ideally the things on your altar will help you to leave behind the stresses of daily life and connect with your inner self in a peaceful way. You might choose photos of inspiring people as well as items that have spiritual significance for you or precious things that people have given you.

3. In planning your altar, think about how you'll use it as well as what you want to have on it. Your altar is a reflection of your life and of your inner self—it is complete when you're happy with the way it looks or how it makes you feel.

One friend has things of nature on her altar because, for her, a feeling of unity comes from being in nature. She has shells, stones, leaves, and branches on her altar, as well as spiritual readings and other things that are meaningful and inspiring to her.

Another friend has her altar at ground level. Her young grandchildren are involved, bringing things that are special to them. This altar is always alive and changing, as some things are removed and others added. The same friend has a small, stuffed Piglet on her altar because Piglet is playful, loving, and devoted—qualities she admires and likes to encourage in herself. Her altar is a joyful place, she says. It cheers her up.

magic wand

TYPE OF ACTIVITY: CRAFT, POSITIVE THOUGHT

Making a magic wand is a playful reminder that you can create your own magic with the power of positive thought and action. When it's done, hang it on the wall or put it where you'll see it often; let it remind you that we always have a choice about our attitudes and the way we look at the world around us. This activity is fun to do with children, who have no trouble believing in magic.

What You Need

• A stick, and things to decorate it with. You can look outside for things of nature, like a branch, feathers, or leaves. You might go to the local hobby shop to buy a plastic stick and colourful decorations like streamers and glitter. Anything goes
• A hot-glue gun and coloured string or ribbon to attach things to the stick
• Acrylic paints and brushes if you plan to paint your stick

How to Make It

1. If you want to paint your stick, do that first.
2. Now glue and tie the decorations onto your magic wand.
3. If you feel uncertain how to go about it, find a girl under the age of eight and ask her to make one with you. She'll show you what to do!
4. When you're done, play with it, dance with it, and then put it where you'll see it often. Bring it down any time you want to make magic.

walking for transformation

TYPE OF ACTIVITY: MOVEMENT, INNER CHANGE

Walking moves the body and deepens the breath; we become relaxed and open to new thoughts and ways of being. Coupled with firm intent, this can provide a wonderful opportunity for inner change. Do this walk when you have a problem, especially if your mind has been turning it over and over with no solution. It can help you shift out of habitual ways of thinking in order to find the answer.

What You Need
• Comfortable walking shoes

How to Do It

1. Plan a distance you're comfortable with; your walk may be around the block or it may be a mile or more.

2. Before you set out, know what you're asking for. You might, for example, have a problem with your boss and want to know how to talk to him or her about it.

3. Be ready to let the problem go and to receive a solution. Be committed to acting on the answer.

4. Begin your walk. You may walk slowly or quickly. Hold a picture of the situation in your mind, but acknowledge that you don't know the answer and let go of active problem solving. The idea is to get your busy mind out of the way so that your creative mind can discover new ways of looking at things. Notice how good it feels to let the problem go. Stay open and let your thoughts come and go; allow them to shift and change and don't hold onto them.

5. Sometime during your walk you may notice a thought that speaks to you a little differently from the others. It may be a sudden, strong new thought. Often it will be a seemingly insignificant thought that keeps coming back until you begin to pay attention to it. If it seems to demand your attention, then pay attention. Keep walking, and ask yourself if this might be the answer, or the beginning of an answer to your question.

6. Sometimes we're given just the beginning of an answer; other times more. One friend says that she doesn't always get an answer, but sometimes a new attitude with which to address the problem. Walk until you feel that you understand what you've been given and are sure you'll remember it after your walk.

7. When you finish walking take some time to become comfortable with your new awareness. Think about how you might act on what you've learned. Write about it in your journal.

letting the body speak

Letting the Body Speak is a tool for self-discovery. Listening to your body helps you get in touch with feelings you don't know you have. It can be especially helpful when you feel a need for self-expression and don't know what you want to express.

Each time you do this exercise you'll find that your listening skills grow. Your body will tell you more, and you'll go deeper into your experience of yourself.

What You Need
- A quiet, private place with room to move

How to Do It
1. Lie on your back on the floor. Quiet your mind, let the demands of the day fall away, and allow yourself to relax.
2. Begin to notice what you're feeling physically in your body. Where is your weight on the floor? Is there any tension in your body? What else do you notice? Don't try to fix anything, just notice.
3. Ask yourself if there is some movement your body wants to make. Is it a stretch? Do you want to curl up in a ball? Maybe just a foot wants to move or maybe just your arm. First imagine the movement and then allow your body to move the way it wants.
4. When you're ready, return to stillness, lying on your back. Notice how the movement has changed you. How is your weight on the floor now? Has the tension in your body changed? What else do you notice?
5. Continue to do this, alternating movement and stillness. Each time, ask how your body wants to move. First imagine the movement and then allow the movement in your body. Your movements may be very small or you may end up standing, crouching, or on all fours.
6. Each time you come back to stillness, notice how you're changed by the movement you made. Where is there tension? Where are you relaxed? Are you warm or cool? Is any part of you tingling? What part of your body is drawing your attention the most?

7. You may begin to notice your emotions as well. Perhaps you're feeling happy or sad, excited, angry, or calm. Accept these feelings, just as you accept the physical feelings. Continue to extend outward with movement and back to stillness. When in stillness, notice how your movement has changed you both physically and emotionally.

8. You may feel that you want to make a sound as you move. Let it come. Sound can allow the primal expression of feelings we don't have words for. As with movement, simply accept it and notice how you feel as you come back to stillness.

9. Words may want to be spoken. Let them come. Accept them, and continue noticing how you feel as you come back to stillness. Continue for as long as you like.

10. At some point you'll notice that you're finished. You may realize that you have no more impulse to move. Perhaps you'll simply know that you're done. When you're ready, get up slowly.

11. Spend some time quietly with yourself. You may feel like drawing or writing about your experience. You may prefer to sit quietly or go for a walk. Give yourself some transition time before returning to normal, daily activities.

your life as a fairy tale

TYPE OF ACTIVITY: WRITING, SELF-DISCOVERY

In telling the story of your life, you can sometimes discover patterns you might otherwise not notice. By telling it as a fairy tale, the door is opened to a vast repertoire of symbolic events and characters. In a fairy tale there is usually a hero, who will meet and overcome challenges. There may be evil, in the form of a king, a witch, or a dragon. Fairy tales allow magic: a young girl is transformed into a bird, a poor man into a rich man, or straw into gold. Anything can happen in a fairy tale.

This activity can be a lot of fun—sometimes lighthearted, sometimes delving deep to bring new understanding or new direction. Remember, you are the main character and this is about exploring your life, not about being a writer. Anything goes, any way that you write it.

What You Need
- Writing materials

How to Do It

1. Spend a few minutes quietly with yourself, letting go of the stresses of the day. When you feel relaxed, begin to think reflectively about your life.

2. Don't try to control your thoughts; just let your mind go where it wants. As you follow your thoughts, you may notice yourself focusing on a particular aspect of your life. It may be a time in the past or in the future, and perhaps a specific area of your life, like relationships or work. If so, stay with this as the subject of your story. If not, then choose an area of your life that you'd like to explore.

3. Focus on the part of your life you will write about. Think about it in terms of fairy tale settings and characters. Where might your story take place? Will it be set in present time or some time in history? Is the location real or fictional? Ask yourself about the people in your story. What roles have they played in your life and how might they be expressed symbolically? What characters will they play in your fairy tale?

4. When you feel ready, start writing. Begin with "Once upon a time . . ." and then keep going. Don't try to control your writing. You may want to change the direction of your story part way through, or you may find yourself writing in free association. Allow yourself to go with whatever happens for you. There are no rules—let the story take you where it wants to go and write for as long as you want.

5. Fairy tales usually have happy endings; however, you may choose to end your story at a sad moment, a moment of learning, or at the end of a chapter. If the story is set in the past, it may end when you get to the present. Any time you want, you can write "The End" or "To Be Continued" and just stop.

6. When you're done, take a short break and then read the story back to yourself. Or, if you'd like to share your fairy tale, invite a friend for tea and read it aloud. What does your story have to tell you about yourself?

a reflective journey

TYPE OF ACTIVITY: INNER JOURNEY

The Reflective Journey follows your life from birth to the present, offering stepping stones of understanding in whatever area you choose to explore.

It works well as a guided visualization, with one person reading it for others to follow. Or guide yourself by reading it onto a tape and then playing it back. (When you read, remember to leave pauses for imagining and reflecting.)

To do the exercise silently on your own, read the instructions and then improvise, following the outline—it doesn't have to be word for word.

What You Need

- A quiet spot where you won't be disturbed
- Optional: cassette tape recorder
- Optional: writing and drawing materials

How to Do It

1. Choose one aspect of your life to explore. On the journey you'll explore your development in this area from birth to the present; for example, the area might be spiritual, career, relationship, or places where you've lived.

2. Lie comfortably on your back. Allow your body to relax and your mind to become quiet as you let go of the outer world and turn your attention inward. Gently bring your attention to the area of your life you have chosen to explore.

3. Imagine yourself standing at the beginning of a path; this represents when you were born. In walking the path you will symbolically move through the years of your life, ending at a vantage point high on a hillside. This will represent where you are now in your life.

4. Begin to walk along the path, noticing what you see and hear around you. Are there birds? Is the sun shining? The path may be steep in some places and gently rising in others. You may find yourself in forest areas or meadows, passing streams or lakes; perhaps you will notice animals along the way.

5. Every so often you'll encounter a memory of a person or an event that has played an important part in your journey. Each memory is a stepping stone from your birth to the present. Stop and spend as much time as you want with each one. With some you may reflect for a while, with others you may move on quickly.

6. When you reach the present you'll find yourself at a vantage point high on the hill. From here you can see far and wide, a panoramic view of the hillside and far beyond. Take time to reflect on your life journey and your experience walking the path. What is the learning, the wisdom that you take from this experience into the next part of your life?

7. Look around for a gift. It might be something of nature—a crystal or a stone, a branch or a flower. Or it might be something that you wouldn't expect to find here. Look around until you find something that speaks to you—this is your gift and a symbol of your learning.

8. When you're ready, leave the hilltop and gently come back to your body and back to the room. Stretch and enjoy the feeling of returning to body awareness.

9. Allow time for reflection before returning to daily activities. You might go for a walk as a symbol of your inner journey and perhaps look for a tangible gift to represent the gift of the hillside. Or you may prefer to sit quietly, perhaps writing about your experience or drawing a picture to represent the journey.

wish tree

TYPE OF ACTIVITY: COLLAGE, VISIONING

Identifying what you want to bring into your life—both tangible and intangible things—can be the first step toward making it happen. A Wish Tree can help you clarify and then stay focused on your goals.

What You Need

- Paper or poster board for the collage
- Magazines suitable to your goals
- Scissors, glue, drawing and colouring materials

How to Do It

1. Draw a tree. It doesn't have to be great art. A child's drawing of a trunk and branches is just right.

2. Look through magazines to find pictures of things you want to bring into your life. It can be tangible things, like a new car, education, or travelling to visit friends and family. Or the pictures can be symbolic of intangible things, like love, friendship, or courage.

3. Glue all the things you want to bring into your life on the branches of your tree. Add any other colouring or decorations that you like.

4. Hang your Wish Tree in a place where you'll see it and be reminded of your goals.

ancestral journey

TYPE OF ACTIVITY: COLLAGE, INNER JOURNEY

The Ancestral Journey allows us to feel the impact of those who came before us, to recognize the support of earlier generations, and to express gratitude for what we have received and how we came to be here. The exercise is written for women, but men can also enjoy this inner journey collage. Simply substitute male names during the exercise; for example, father and grandfather instead of mother and grandmother.

What You Need

- Paper or poster board for the collage
- Magazines suitable to your subject
- Scissors, glue, drawing and colouring materials

How to Do It

1. Sit or lie in a comfortable position and let the stress of the day fall away as you relax and get ready to spend some special time with yourself.

2. Spend a few minutes thinking of the women in your family—your daughters, yourself, your mother, your grandmother, and your great grandmother, if you knew her. Imagine the generations of women lining up, with the youngest in the front and the oldest in the back. Visualize the line slightly on the diagonal so that you can see them all, slightly behind and beside each other.

3. Look for your connection to all the women in your history, the ways in which each woman behind you is supporting you to be who you are today. Negative thoughts may come first. Think about how even your negative history has had a hand in shaping and strengthening you. Be with all that comes up. Gently persist until you also see the positive—the love and the support offered by the generations that have come before you.

4. Look forward toward the younger ones. You may not have daughters. Are there other young women with whom you interact as teacher, aunt, or friend? Experience the support of your ancestors moving through you in the love and support you offer the generations of women that come after you.

5. Now look through magazines and cut out images for your collage. Your images may be representational or completely symbolic. You may represent your grandmother with a picture of an older woman who happens to have a similar smile, or you may represent her with a picture of a computer or a paintbrush. You may not know why you're choosing certain pictures. Just follow your intuition. Don't think about how they will fit together; choose anything that feels right to you for any reason.

6. Arrange the images on your paper and move them around until you like the way it looks. When you have it the way you want it, glue the images in place. Add drawing or colouring if you like.

7. When you're done, spend time in reflection. You might write in your journal, or talk to a friend about what you learned.

> If you're adopted, this might be a journey of your adoptive family, your birth family (if you know about them), or both.

full-body collage

Making a collage of your own body is an introspective process and can be illuminating. It can deepen your knowledge of yourself, where you are in your life, and how you got there; it can also help to define new direction.

This project is fun to share with a friend. If you do it alone, ask someone to help you draw your body shape before you begin. Set aside a morning or afternoon—this is a leisurely process and it's better not to rush it.

What You Need
- A large sheet of paper, big enough for your full-size body shape
- Craft items such as glitter, ribbon, yarn, or bits of fabric
- A basket or bag for collecting things on your nature walk
- Magazines for cutting out pictures and words
- Scissors, glue, tape, and painting or colouring materials

How to Do It
1. First, take turns drawing your body shapes. Have one person lie down on the paper while the other draws around the shape of the body. Cut out your body shape and set it aside.
2. Lie comfortably on your back, quiet your mind, and allow yourself to relax. Take a few minutes to think about your body. Think about how it has been at different times in your life; remember climbing trees, playing soccer, or birthing babies. Think about the parts of your body that you're happy with, and the parts that you don't like. Think about how it supports you in doing all the things of daily life that you take for granted. You live in your body; it is your first and last home and is always with you. Take a moment to appreciate it.
3. Now take a walk outside looking for things of nature to include in your collage. If you live in the city, perhaps there's a park nearby or maybe your own backyard will have treasures waiting for you. There doesn't have to be a logical reason for choosing the things you find. If it draws you, put it in your basket or bag.
4. When you get back from your walk, look through magazines for pictures to add to your collection of treasures.

5. Begin to arrange things on your body shape. You may have reasons for putting things in certain places or you may not know why things go where they go. Take your time and decorate your body any way you like. Use glue and tape to secure things in place and add colouring or painting if you wish. Collect more objects or pictures and add those too. There are no rules.

6. If you do the project with a friend, take turns showing each other your collages when you have finished. Talk about your collage and the process of making it. If you're alone, write about it in your journal. Hang it on the wall where you'll see it often.

mandala

TYPE OF ACTIVITY: DRAWING, COLOURING, SELF-EXPLORATION

A mandala is a symmetrical design that uses shape and colour to express an idea. Mandalas are usually abstract, sometimes geometric, and often, but not necessarily, circular. Your personal mandala represents the layers of your self, from the innermost self outward to the face you show the world, with all the protective layers in between. The relationship mandala is an extension of the personal mandala and can illuminate aspects of a relationship in a new way. It can be done for any relationship between family members, friends, or co-workers.

What You Need
- Drawing paper
- Materials for colouring. Colour is important in a mandala; oil pastels are great because they have strong, vibrant colour. Felt pens are also good

How to Make a Personal Mandala
1. Sit or lie comfortably with your eyes closed as you let the demands of daily life fall away. Allow yourself to relax. Let go of the outer world and turn your attention inward.
2. Now imagine your innermost self, the part of you that is most hidden from the world. What do you notice about this inner you? Stay with your sense of self, noticing anything that comes up, until you feel ready to begin drawing.
3. Begin your mandala in the centre of the page, using colour and shape symbolically to represent your innermost self. The size of this representation is up to you, and will probably be different for every person. Choose colours and shapes that feel right to you. You don't have to know why you are choosing them. And remember, this is not about making art.
4. Gradually move outward from the centre of the page, allowing your colours and shapes to represent each protective layer of your inner self. When you reach the outside edges of your mandala, depict the face that you show to the world.
5. When you look at your finished mandala, you'll see yourself from a new perspective. This is who you are in colour. What do you learn about yourself from the colours and shapes you've chosen?

How to Make a Relationship Mandala

1. In this exercise you make two mandalas on the same page. The first is your personal mandala. The second is for the other person. Let the mandalas come from inside, where you intuitively know about this relationship. Don't try to control them.

2. When you're done, have a look at the page. What does it have to tell you? Colour, size, placement on the page, kind of lines (soft or sharp edges)—all these things can tell you something about the relationship. Is one mandala big and the other small? Is one crowding into the other's space? There is no right or wrong way to interpret your drawing—you may have reasons for your interpretation or simply a feeling about what it means. Let yourself be intuitive as you look at the mandalas and how they interact on the page.

love letter to yourself

TYPE OF ACTIVITY: WRITING, APPRECIATING YOURSELF

A love letter is a heartwarming and supportive view of ourselves as someone else sees us. By stepping out of habitual ways of looking at ourselves we can create this kind of loving support for ourselves.

What You Need
- Writing materials

How to Do It

1. Write a letter acknowledging something positive about yourself; write as though it comes from someone else.

2. Acknowledge yourself for something you've done well, for a positive quality you've developed or a virtue you feel successful with. You can write about something you're still working on, as if you're good at it already, or say how much you have improved in an area. Be in love with yourself and write from the heart.

3. Sign it with your own name or from a secret admirer. Put it in an envelope and mail it to yourself.

virtues exploration

TYPE OF ACTIVITY: WRITING, SELF-ACKNOWLEDGEMENT, SELF-IMPROVEMENT
The development of virtues, or positive qualities, is an important part of self-development. The Virtues Exploration can help you focus on qualities you want to work on as well as acknowledge what you're already good at. It can be fun and supportive to do this exercise with a friend.

What You Need
- Writing materials

How to Do It
1. Make a list of as many virtues as you can think of. Include anything that you think of as a positive quality. Kindness and honesty are commonly thought of as virtues, but what about courage, creativity, and joyfulness?

2. Read over the list and pick out the ones you think you're good at. These are the ways in which you act positively in your life; things that make you feel good about yourself. Write them down, and beside each one say why you think you're good at it. For example, "I'm good at honesty, because I always keep my promises" or "Last week I was good at flexibility when our camping trip was rained out and we unexpectedly had to make other plans."

3. Now choose one that you need to work on—something that you want to practise for your own self-development. Write it down, and beside it write why you think you aren't good at it. For example, if you chose impatience you might say, "I'm impatient whenever anyone is late" or "I feel impatient when the children spill things or make messes."

4. Think of several ways you could work on developing this virtue during the following week. Using the above examples, you might decide to practise breathing deeply and relaxing when someone is late (since there's probably nothing you can do about it!) or to be more understanding with your children when they make mistakes. Make a commitment to doing these things.

5. At the end of the week ask yourself how you did. If you did the exercise with a friend, talk about it together.

virtues acknowledgement

TYPE OF ACTIVITY: HONOURING OTHERS

To be recognized for the positive qualities we display in our lives is supportive and validating. To be honoured this way at a special occasion makes us feel especially appreciated. The Virtues Acknowledgement is a card given on an occasion like a birthday, Christmas, or Valentine's Day.

What You Need

- Poster board or drawing paper, 8 1/2 x 11 inches or larger
- A photo of the person being honoured
- Felt pens
- Glue

How to Do It

1. At the top of your card, glue a photo of the person to be honoured and put his or her name beside it.
2. Below the picture make a separate place for each person to write an acknowledgement. Choose from the ideas below or make up your own.
3. Have everyone write on the card ahead of time so that it will be ready for the special occasion. People can choose to sign their acknowledgements or be anonymous.

For a birthday card, draw balloons—one for each person who will sign the card. Each balloon should be big enough for someone to write his or her acknowledgement inside. Put strings on the balloons and tie them together at the bottom of the page with a ribbon.

At Christmas, draw tree ornaments—as many as there are people to sign the card and big enough for them to write in. If you use a large poster board you might draw a tree and hang the ornaments on the tree.

For Valentine's Day, draw a big heart for each person to write in. Arrange the hearts in a bouquet, like flowers or balloons. Decorate the rest of the page with small hearts.

fragrant flower facial

Guests at our Women's Weekends are treated to a Sunday morning facial. It's a relaxing experience and can be enjoyed by men as well as women. You can give yourself this facial, or you and a friend can treat each other. Your face will feel warm and radiant and you'll look relaxed, fresh, and beautiful.

Getting Ready

- Read the instructions before beginning to make and gather the things you need.
- If you plan to make your own calendula cream, note that the flower petals must soak in oil for two weeks before making the cream. (Once it's made, however, you'll have enough for many facials.) You can also buy calendula cream in most natural food stores.
- We use fresh organic ingredients whenever possible. If fresh herbs and flowers aren't available you can use dried ones, available at many natural food stores.
- Prepare the scrub, cream, toner, and moisturizer following the recipes given below.
- For the Lavender Steam you'll need 1/2 cup of lavender flowers.
- You'll need three bowls: one large one (bigger around than your face for the Lavender Steam), and two small bowls, one for mixing the Almond Oatmeal Scrub and one for mixing the clay mask.
- For the clay mask you'll need 3 tablespoons of Bentonite clay (found at most natural food stores). *Please note that you shouldn't use a clay mask if your skin is very dry or delicate.*
- You'll also need two cotton balls, two towels, a washcloth, and something to hold your hair off your face.
- Finally, you'll need a kettle or something else to boil water in.

If you're doing this with a friend:
- Prepare a comfortable place where the person receiving the facial can lie down, and where you can sit at her head to give the facial.
- Double everything in your preparations, except for the cream, toner, and moisturizer.

Preparing Products for the Facial

Almond Oatmeal Scrub

• Place 1/4 cup organic oats and 1/8 cup almonds in a blender or food processor and process to a fine, granular consistency. If you make a larger quantity it will keep well in a jar in the freezer.

Calendula Cream

If your skin is oily you won't use this cream for the facial, although it can be used as a general skin cream for any part of the body. If you don't use the cream you'll need a small amount of unroasted sesame oil to protect the skin around your eyes and lips during the mask.

1. In a clean jar, soak 1/2 cup calendula flowers in 1 cup of unroasted sesame oil. Let it sit in natural light for two weeks, in the sun if possible. Shake the jar every day, making sure the oil covers all the flowers.

2. After two weeks strain the oil from the flowers, squeezing the flowers to get all the oil. Simmer the oil in a saucepan with 3 tablespoons beeswax until the beeswax is melted. Allow it to cool to room temperature.

3. Place this mixture in a blender with 1/2 tablespoon vegetable glycerine. Blend slowly while adding 1/2 cup pure aloe vera gel. Keep blending until the mixture is smooth and creamy. It should have a fairly thick consistency.

4. You can add a few drops of Vitamin E oil, or any essential oil, if you like.

5. This recipe makes a generous amount of cream. Use it as a daily skin cream for any skin type. It keeps well—we once kept some in a glass jar on a windowsill for 11 months and it was still good. In the fridge it would keep longer.

6. Calendula is soothing, cleansing, and said to be antiseptic, anti-fungal, and anti-inflammatory. Calendula and aloe vera gel are both said to regenerate cells and heal tissue.

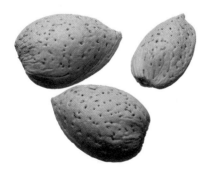

Chamomile-Sage Toner

• Place 1 tablespoon chamomile and 4 or 5 sage leaves in a bowl and pour 1 cup fresh, boiled water over them. Cool and strain.

• This toner will keep in the fridge for about a week. Leftover toner can be put in your bath or used to water the plants.

Rose-Honey Moisturizer

• Place 3 tablespoons rose petals and 1/4 teaspoon honey in a bowl and pour 1 cup fresh, boiled water over them. Cool and strain.

• This moisturizer also keeps in the fridge for about a week. It's a fragrant addition to a bath and can be used to water plants.

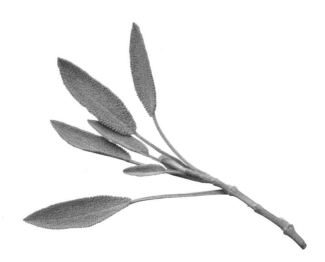

How to Do the Facial

STEP ONE: THE LAVENDER STEAM

• Place 1/2 cup of lavender flowers in a large bowl and pour about 4 cups of boiling water over the flowers. Hold your face over the bowl and cover your head with a towel to capture the steam. Stay in the steam until you feel it starting to cool down. Pat your face dry.

STEP TWO: THE ALMOND-OATMEALSCRUB

• Mix 4 tablespoons of Almond Oatmeal Scrub with a bit of warm water; use just enough water to make it creamy. Using your fingers, gently scrub your face—and your neck if you like—with this mixture. Rinse with lukewarm water and pat dry.

STEP THREE: PROTECTING YOUR
EYES AND LIPS

This step isn't needed if you don't do the clay mask.

• With your baby finger or a cotton swab apply a very small bit of Calendula Cream or unroasted sesame oil under your eyes and on the eyelids. In the same way, apply some cream around the outside of your lips. This will replenish natural oils in the skin and keep delicate areas moist during the clay mask.

STEP FOUR: MASSAGING YOUR FACE

· Using the tips of your index, middle, and ring fingers, and beginning in the middle of your forehead, massage very gently in a circular motion, working your way to the outside of your forehead. Continue all the way down the sides of your face until your hands meet at your chin.

· Massage up your cheeks to the cheekbones, follow the cheekbones to the nose, and massage around the nose with tiny circular motions.

· Place a thumb under each eyebrow and gently press in and upwards along the length of the eyebrows. In the same way, begin at the inside corner of each eye and press gently with your middle fingers along the underside of the eyes.

· With your thumbs or middle fingers, press gently above your eyebrows from the inside edges of the eyebrows to the outside of your forehead.

· Massage inside the ears with one finger. Squeeze the ear lobe and all the way up and around the ear.

· Now use all your fingers to massage the scalp in a circular motion. This can be more vigorous.

· Finish by gently tapping the tips of the fingers across the whole face, and then rest for a moment.

STEP FIVE: THE CLAY MASK

If your skin is very dry, delicate, or sensitive, don't do this step.

· Mix 3 tablespoons of the Bentonite clay powder with enough warm water to make a paste. Use your fingers to apply the paste to your face, leaving a small area clear around your lips and eyes. No clay should go between your cheekbones and your eyes, and none under your eyebrows.

· Apply a thick layer in areas with large pores or oily skin. Don't use clay in areas with dry skin or visible delicate blood vessels.

· As soon as it dries, remove the clay mask gently with warm water and a washcloth. Rinse your face and pat dry.

STEP SIX: CHAMOMILE-SAGE TONER

· Soak a cotton swab with toner and apply it to your face and neck. Apply until your face is dripping wet and then pat dry. This toner restores the pH balance of the skin after the clay mask.

STEP SEVEN: ROSE-HONEY MOISTURIZER

· Take a fresh cotton swab, soak it with moisturizer, and apply it to your face and neck. Again, apply until your face is dripping wet and then pat dry.

STEP EIGHT: CALENDULA CREAM

If your skin is oily, don't do this step.

· Apply this fragrant flower cream to your face and neck with gentle upward strokes.

resources and further reading

Yoga Philosophy

Baba Hari Dass. *Ashtanga Yoga Primer.* Santa Cruz, CA: Sri Rama Publishing, 1981.

Baba Hari Dass. *Everyday Peace, Letters for Life.* Santa Cruz, CA: Sri Rama Publishing, 2000.

Baba Hari Dass. *The Path to Enlightenment Is Not a Highway.* Santa Cruz, CA: Sri Rama Publishing, 1996.

Baba Hari Dass. *Silence Speaks.* Santa Cruz, CA: Sri Rama Publishing, 1997.

Baba Hari Dass. *Yoga Sutras of Patanjali: A Study Guide for Book 1.* Santa Cruz, CA: Sri Rama Publishing, 1999.

Swami Prabhavananda and Christopher Isherwood, translation and commentary. *How to Know God: The Yoga Aphorisms of Patanjali.* 1953, Reprint Hollywood: Vedanta Press, 1987.

Note: *The profits from the sale of Baba Hari Dass's books are used directly to support Shri Ram Orphanage in India. Founded by Baba Hari Dass, Shri Ram provides a loving home for needy and orphaned children. Shri Ram's school and free medical clinic serve these children as well as families of nearby villages. For further information, please contact Sri Rama foundation, PO Box 2550, Santa Cruz, California, 95063.*

Related Buddhist Writing

Beck, Charlotte Joko. *Everyday Zen: Love and Work.* New York: Harper Collins, 1989.

Boorstein, Sylvia. *It's Easier Than You Think.* New York: Harper Collins, 1997.

Chodron, Pema. *When Things Fall Apart: Heart Advice for Difficult Times.* Boston: Shambhala Publications, 2000.

Rinpoche, Sogyal. *The Tibetan Book of Living and Dying.* San Francisco: Harper San Francisco, 1994.

Developing Positive Qualities

Kavelin-Popov, Linda. *The Virtues Project: Educator's Guide.* Carson: Jalmar Press, 2000.

Kavelin-Popov, Linda. *The Family Virtues Guide.* New York: Plume, 1997.

Asanas

Baba Hari Dass. *Ashtanga Yoga Primer.*

Santa Cruz, CA: Sri Rama Publishing, 1981.

Couch, Jean. *The Runner's Yoga Book.* Berkeley: Rodmell Press, 1990.

Lasater, Judith. *Relax and Renew.* Berkeley: Rodmell Press, 1995.

Mehta, Mira. *How to Use Yoga. Acropolis Books.* First published in 1994 Lorenz Books.

Stewart, Mary and K. Phillips. *Yoga Over 50.* New York: Simon & Schuster, 1993.

Asana Product Sources

Metaphysical book and gift shops sometimes carry the more common yoga props like mats, bolsters, and eye pillows.

Halfmoon Yoga Props Ltd.
877-731-7099
www.halfmoonyogaprops.com

Ayurveda

Chopra, Deepak. *Perfect Health.* New York: Three Rivers Press, 2001.

Lad, Dr. Visant. *The Complete Book of Ayurvedic Home Remedies.* New York: Three Rivers Press, 1998.

Morningstar, Amadea. *The Ayurvedic Cookbook.* Twin Lakes, WI: Lotus Press, 1990.

Godagama, Dr. Shantha. *The Handbook of Ayurveda.* Boston: Charles E. Tuttle & Co, 1996.

Everyday Ayurveda
PO Box 681
Cedar Ridge, CA 95924
(530) 470-9789
www.everydayayurveda.org
A non-profit agency with a comprehensive listing of Ayurvedic teachers, practitioners, and schools, as well as businesses that provide Ayurvedic products and services.

Ayurveda Product Sources

Bazaar of India Imports
1810 University Avenue
Berkeley, CA 94703-1516
800-261-7662
(510) 549-9990
www.bazaarofindia.com

Lotus Herbs
620 Cabrillo Avenue
Santa Cruz, CA 95065
(831) 479-1667
herbs@lotusayurveda.com
www.lotusayurveda.com

index

recipe index